Patient-Reported Outcomes in Performance Measurement

David Cella, Elizabeth A. Hahn,
Sally E. Jensen, Zeeshan Butt, Cindy J. Nowinski,
Nan Rothrock, Kathleen N. Lohr

RTI Press

The RTI Press mission is to disseminate information about RTI research, analytic tools, and technical expertise to a national and international audience. RTI Press publications are peer-reviewed by at least two independent substantive experts and one or more Press editors.

RTI International is an independent, nonprofit research organization dedicated to improving the human condition by turning knowledge into practice. RTI offers innovative research and technical services to governments and businesses worldwide in the areas of health and pharmaceuticals, education and training, surveys and statistics, advanced technology, international development, economic and social policy, energy and the environment, and laboratory testing and chemistry services.

Library of Congress Control Number: 2015948921

ISBN 978-1-934831-14-4
(refers to printed version)

RTI Press publication No. BK-0014-1509
doi:http://dx.doi.org/10.3768/rtipress.2015.bk.0014.1509

This publication is part of the RTI Press Book series.
RTI International
3040 East Cornwallis Road, PO Box 12194
Research Triangle Park, NC 27709-2194 USA
rtipress@rti.org
www.rti.org

Contents

(continued)

Contents (continued)

Tables

Figure

Introduction

The increasing integration of health care delivery systems provides an opportunity to manage entire episodes of care in a patient-focused manner and to assess the impact of care on patient outcomes, including *patient-reported outcomes* (PROs).[1] The National Institutes of Health (NIH) PROMIS initiative (for Patient Reported Outcomes Measurement Information System) describes PROs as direct feedback from patients "on their feelings or what they are able to do as they are dealing with chronic diseases or conditions." They reflect the health status or health-related quality of life circumstances of patients (broadly defined). Such information is reported by individuals themselves or, in some cases, by proxy respondents such as parents for young children or close relatives of persons unable to report for themselves.

PRO information is widely gathered in clinical and health services research; it is increasingly collected and used in clinical practice settings as well.[2-7] PROs are relevant for many activities: helping patients and their clinicians make informed decisions about health care, monitoring the progress of care, setting policies for coverage and reimbursement of health services, improving the quality of health care services, and tracking or reporting on the performance of health care delivery organizations.

These last two activities are gaining increasing attention in the US health care system. The nation is engaging in more efforts to expand health care coverage to many millions of citizens through the Patient Protection and Affordable Care Act (ACA). Many organizations are working to ensure higher value of health care through enhanced attention to measuring and improving quality of care and patient outcomes.[8] For example, the Patient-Centered Outcomes Research Institute (PCORI), established by the ACA, is actively pursuing ways to increase the use of PROs for clinical care, research, and performance assessment.

The National Quality Forum Project

The National Quality Forum (NQF), a national organization that has been deeply involved in moving the quality-improvement agenda forward for many years (http://www.qualityforum.org), endorses and promulgates quality-of-care and performance measures that various provider groups, regulatory agencies, payers and insurers, and others can use for accountability and quality improvement activities. In 2012 and 2013, the organization began an initiative to find PROs that might be added to its extensive collection of performance measures. Its *National Voluntary Consensus Standards for Patient Outcomes: A Consensus Report* defined outcomes as being important because they "reflect the reason that an individual seeks healthcare services."[1] The individual patient's voice in many performance measures, however, has largely been missing. Few ways to assess performance are available at the organizational level, even though patients are often the best able to report on the experiences and results of their individual care.

To fill that gap, NQF convened an expert panel at two public meetings and, as background for its deliberations, commissioned two authoritative background papers. This monograph is a revised and updated version of the first of these two papers, which provided the background on issues about selecting PROs for use in a variety of applications pertinent to the NQF mission and activities. The second paper, *Patient-Reported Outcomes in Performance Measurement*,[9] dealt with issues relating to processes for endorsing performance measures that reflect the end results (ultimate outcomes) of health care. Its primary focus was on accountable health care organizations.

This monograph applies the conceptual and organizational frameworks that NQF has pioneered in the past decade or so. NQF distinguishes PROs, patient-reported outcome measures (or PROMs), and patient-reported outcome performance measures (or PRO-PMs). NQF endorses PRO-PMs through transparent and consensus-based procedures. This monograph addresses the PROs that are likely to be used to inform PRO measures (PROMs) that would underpin scientifically acceptable and feasible performance measures. We do not address issues with identifying, evaluating, or endorsing PRO-PMs for health care organizations or clinicians.

To accomplish our assigned objective, we completed a comprehensive review of the published peer-reviewed literature as well as published documents (e.g., book chapters, position statements; guidance from the US Food and Drug Administration[10]) about standard measurement theory. Based on our findings in the published literature, we created a comprehensive annotated outline reflecting the methodological considerations most important to address. We then revised it in consultation with representatives from NQF to ensure that the paper accomplished the NQF's high-priority objectives.

Following the initial drafting of the manuscript, our group of authors at Northwestern University worked in conjunction with Kathleen Lohr, RTI International, who comprehensively reviewed and revised the manuscript draft. We submitted the revised manuscript draft for review and comment at the NQF Patient Reported Outcomes Workshop 1 in July 2012. A final version of the manuscript, which incorporated revisions based on feedback from the workshop, was submitted to NQF in September 2012. That manuscript includes numerous authoritative citations to research from this field up through that date. Dr. Lohr and the other authors revised the manuscript further to meet the requirements of an RTI Press monograph and to update some of the citations; the result is this monograph.

Concepts and Definitions

PROs are defined here as any report of the status of a patient's health condition, health behavior, or experience with health care that comes directly from the patient, without interpretation of the patient's response by a clinician or anyone else (Table 1). There are many available PRO measurement tools, which we refer to here as patient-reported outcome measures, or PROMs. By using direct, unfiltered inquiry, PROMs measure what patients are able to do and how they feel. They reflect the direct voice of the patient, as perceived by the patient.

Table 1. Definitions and key concepts for patient-reported outcomes and measures

Key Concept	Definition
Patient	A person who is receiving health care services or using long-term health care support services.
Patient-reported outcome (PRO)	Any information on the outcomes of health care obtained directly from patients without modification by clinicians or other health care professionals. For purposes of this monograph, we use this term broadly to include any patient input, whether or not it is standardized or gathered with a structured questionnaire.
Patient-reported outcome measure (PROM)	Any standardized or structured questionnaire regarding the status of a patient's health condition, health behavior, or experience with health care that comes directly from the patient (i.e., a PRO). The use of a structured, standardized tool such as a PROM will yield quantitative data that enables comparison of patient groups or providers. One example of a PROM is the nine-item Patient Health Questionnaire (PHQ-9).
Performance measure	Numeric quantification of health care quality for a designated accountable health care entity, such as a hospital, health plan, nursing home, clinician, etc.
PRO-based performance measure (PRO-PM)	A performance measure that is based on patient-reported outcomes assessed through data often collected through a PROM and then aggregated for an accountable health care entity. One example is the percentage of patients in an accountable care organization with an improved depression score as measured by a standardized tool such as the PHQ-9.
e-health	Health-related Internet applications that deliver a range of content, connectivity, and clinical care. Examples include online formularies, prescription refills, test results, physician-patient communication.[11,12]
Patient-centered outcomes research (PCOR)	Integration of patient perspectives and experiences with clinical and biological data collected from the patient to evaluate the safety and efficacy of an intervention (www.pcori.org).
Reliability	The extent to which a scale or measure yields reproducible and consistent results.[13] Reliability of data elements refers to repeatability and reproducibility of the data elements for the same population in the same time period. Reliability of the measure score refers to the proportion of variation in the performance scores attributable to systematic differences across the measured entities (or signal) in relation to random error (or noise).
Validity	The extent to which an instrument measures what it is intended to measure and can be useful for its intended purpose.[13] Validity of instruments can be assessed in numerous ways, often in comparison with an authoritative source (such as a similar validated instrument). Validity of measure scores can refer to the correctness of conclusions that users might draw from a reliable and valid instrument (as, for instance, that a better score on a quality measure reflects higher quality of health care).

Using Patient-Reported Outcome Measures (PROMs)

A large literature supports the use of PROMs and provides cogent evidence suggesting that clinicians are limited in accurately estimating outcomes for patients.[14-18] PROMs enable clinicians, patients and families, and others to assess patient-reported health status domains (e.g., health status; physical, mental, and social functioning; health behavior; experience with health care). A wide variety of patient-level instruments to measure PROMs have been used for clinical research purposes and to guide clinical care. Many have been evaluated and catalogued by the NIH PROMIS network and made available through the PROMIS Assessment Center (www.nihpromis.org/software/assessmentcenter).

Two major challenges to using PROMs for purposes of accountability and performance improvement must be addressed. First, they have not yet been widely adopted in clinical use; thus, they are unfamiliar to many health care professionals, payers, and others in health care systems. Second, little is known about the best set of responsive questions to aggregate for the purpose of measuring *performance* of the health care organizations and systems.

Many in the health sector are showing increasing interest in moving toward use of PROMs for these clinical, quality improvement, and accountability applications. Foundational work still needs to address methodological and data challenges. Efforts in the early 2010s focused on developing and testing mechanisms for collecting patient-reported data. A crucial element of this is considering methodological issues in some depth. Among the more difficult problems are collecting PRO data in the clinical environment and aggregating data to assess organization- and clinician-level performance.

In the remainder of this monograph, we address the major methodological issues related to the selection, administration, and use of PROMs for individual patients in clinical practice settings. We highlight best practices in identifying and using PROMs in performance measures. Given such information, those concerned with identifying and choosing appropriate PROMs as candidate measures for use in performance assessment and related applications can move ahead in this arena.

Types of Patient-Reported Outcomes

PROMs can be used to assess a wide variety of health-relevant concepts. Of particular salience for quality and performance measurement efforts are the following five categories: health-related quality of life, functional status, symptoms and symptom burden, health behaviors, and the patient's health care experience. These concepts are neither mutually exclusive nor exhaustive.

Table 2 summarizes the main characteristics of these types of PROMs. In the table, we highlight only key advantages or drawbacks for each PRO category. In the subsections that follow, we focus on core components or attributes of the specific category in question of particular relevance for measurement (including efficient performance measurement). Consequently, the information for any given PRO category may differ from that for other categories.

Table 2. Main characteristics of patient-reported outcomes

PRO Category	Main Characteristics	Main Strengths	Main Limitations
Health-related quality of life (HRQL)	• Is multidimensional • Can be generic or condition-specific	• Yields a global summary of well-being	• May not be considered a sufficiently specific construct
Functional status	• Reflects ability to perform specific activities	• Can be used in addition to performance-based measures of function	• May reflect variations in self-reported capability and actual performance of activities
Symptoms and symptom burden	• Are specific to type of symptom of interest • May identify symptoms not otherwise captured by medical workup	• Are best assessed through self-report	• May fail to capture general, global aspects of well-being considered important to patients

(continued)

Table 2. Main characteristics of patient-reported outcomes *(continued)*

PRO Category	Main Characteristics	Main Strengths	Main Limitations
Health behaviors	• Are specific to type of behavior • Typically measure frequency of behavior	• Target specific behavior categories	• Validity may be affected by social desirability • May produce potential patient discomfort in reporting socially undesirable behaviors
Patient experience	• Concerns satisfaction with health care delivery, treatment recommendations, and medications (or other therapies) • Reflects actual experiences with health care services • Fosters patient activation	• Is an essential component of patient-centered care • Is valued by patients, families, and policy makers • Relates to treatment adherence • Relates to health behaviors and health outcomes	• May be a complex, multidimensional construct • Requires confidentiality to ensure patient comfort in disclosing negative experiences • Does not provide sufficient evidence that activation enhances health care decision making

Health-Related Quality of Life

One class of PRO measures health-related quality of life (HRQL). HRQL is a multidimensional[19] construct encompassing physical, social, and emotional well-being associated with illness and its treatment.[20] Different types of HRQL measures[21,22] are useful for different purposes.[23] Numerous generic health status measures, such as the Medical Outcomes Study Short Form SF-36 (and related measures) and the Sickness Impact Profile are classic examples.[24–27] This type of PROM is useful in assessing individuals both with and without a health condition. Such data allow researchers, clinicians, and others to compare groups with and without a specific condition and to estimate population norms.

A health utility or preference measure is also not disease-specific. It provides a score ranging from 0 (death) to 1 (perfect health) that represents the value that a patient places on his or her own health.[28] Experts can use scores from these types of measures to calculate quality-adjusted life years or compare information to population norms.

Many PROMs are intended for use in populations with chronic illnesses.[29-31] Over the past 8 years, the PROMIS network has developed a considerable number of PROMs in physical, mental, and social health for adults and infants, children, and adolescents with chronic conditions.[32,33] Neuro-QOL is another measurement effort focused on capturing important areas of functioning and well-being in neurologic diseases.[34] These measurement efforts do not reference a specific disease in the items; thus, they permit comparisons across conditions.

Other PROMs are targeted on a specific disease (e.g., spinal cord injury) or treatment (e.g., chemotherapy).[35,36] Often these instruments are developed so that investigators can demonstrate responsiveness to treatment in a clinical trial rather than compare data against population norms or information on other conditions.[37] Condition-specific PROMs often provide additional, complementary information about a patient's HRQL.[30,38-40]

Functional Status

Another type of PROM is a functional status measure. Functional status refers to a patient's ability to perform both basic and more advanced (instrumental) activities of daily life.[41] Examples of functional status include physical function, cognitive function, and sexual function. As with HRQL instruments, a large number of functional status measures exist, but they vary widely in quality.[42] Some may address a very specific type of function (e.g., Upper Limb Functional Index) or be developed for use in a specific disease population (e.g., patients with multiple sclerosis), whereas others may be appropriate for use across chronic conditions.[43-49]

Symptoms and Symptom Burden

Symptoms such as fatigue and pain intensity are key domains for PROMs. Symptoms are typically negative, and their presence and intensity are best assessed through patient report.[50] Scales characterize the severity of the symptoms. The impact of symptoms, such as the degree to which pain interferes with usual functioning, is also a common focus of PROMs. Symptom burden captures the combination of both symptom severity and impact experienced with a specific disease or treatment.[50]

Common symptom and symptom burden measures include the Functional Assessment of Chronic Illness Therapy—Fatigue scale, which is not targeted on any one condition. By contrast, disease-focused symptom indexes include the symptom indexes for various cancer types set out by the National Comprehensive Cancer Network and a dyspnea-specific instrument for chronic obstructive pulmonary disease.[51,52] PROMIS investigators developed the PROMIS Pain Interference measure, which quantifies the impact of pain on functioning.[53]

Health Behaviors

Yet another category of PROMs assesses health behaviors. Although health behaviors may be considered predictors of health outcomes, they are also health outcomes in their own right in the sense that health care interventions can have an impact on them. Information from health behavior PROMs serves several important clinical purposes. Clinicians can use it to monitor risk behaviors with potentially deleterious health consequences. This information enables practitioners to identify areas for risk reduction and health promotion interventions among their patients. Health behavior PROMs can also be used to assess patients' response to health promotion interventions and to monitor health behaviors over time.

Health risk assessments (HRAs) illustrate how health behavior PROMs can be incorporated into health promotion and disease prevention programs. Defined by the US Centers for Disease Control and Prevention (CDC) as tools to measure individual health, HRAs may consist of clinical examination or laboratory test results as well as health behavior PROMs.[54] A recent report from the US Agency for Healthcare Research and Quality (AHRQ) identified three key components in the process of implementing HRAs in health promotion: (1) patient self-reported information to identify risk factors for disease, (2) individualized health-specific feedback to patients based upon the information they reported, and (3) at least one health promotion recommendation or intervention.[55]

Although HRAs have been implemented in community settings, universities, and health maintenance organizations, they have been most commonly implemented in workplace settings.[55] An extensive review of HRA program outcomes concluded that, in many cases, implementing HRA programs improved health behaviors and intermediate health outcomes (e.g., blood pressure); however, the evidence did not demonstrate whether using HRAs affected disease incidence or health outcomes over the medium to long term.[55]

As the emphasis on the importance of health behaviors has increased, so has the number of available PROs developed to assess health behaviors across multiple domains. Health behavior PROs may assess general health by measuring risk factors without a focus on a specific disease or behavioral category. Two examples of health behavior PROMs measuring multiple risk factors that the National Committee for Quality Assurance has certified are the Personal Wellness Profile[56] and the Insight Health Risk Appraisal Survey.[57]

In addition, several large-scale health behavior assessment systems provide additional context for the use of general health behavior PROMs. The Behavioral Risk Factor Surveillance System (BRFSS), created in 1984 by the CDC as a state-based system, uses a standardized questionnaire to measure health risk and health promotion behaviors. These include health awareness, tobacco use, consumption of fruits and vegetables, physical activity, seatbelt use, immunization, and alcohol consumption.[58] The National Health and Nutrition Examination Survey (NHANES) constitutes another large-scale implementation of health behavior PROMs. Established by the CDC in the 1960s, NHANES includes health behavior surveys in addition to clinical examinations to assess health status at the population level.[59]

The health behavior survey portion of NHANES assesses a wide range of health risk and health promotion behaviors, including smoking, drug use, alcohol use, sexual practices, physical activity, dietary intake, and reproductive health practices.[59] Health behavior PROMs can also assess risk factors associated with specific diseases (e.g., smoking) or those related to specific behavioral categories (e.g., physical activity, seatbelt use, food consumption). The health risk survey, an interactive computer-based survey assessing alcohol consumption and smoking,[60] is one example. Another is the CAGE-Adapted to Include Drugs (CAGE-AID) questionnaire, a self-reported screening measure of substance use disorder among treatment-seeking adolescents. Its name derives from its four main questions (Cutting down, being Annoyed if people criticize drinking, feeling Guilty about drinking, and needing an Eye-opener).[61]

A subset of health behavior PROMs assesses health-promoting behaviors. Examples of such PROM instruments include "Starting the conversation," a brief measure of dietary intake;[62] "Exercise as the fifth vital sign," a brief measure of physical activity;[63] School Health Action, Planning and Evaluation System (SHAPES), a school-based self-report physical activity measure;[64] and the Morisky Medication Adherence Scale (8-item).[65]

Patient Experience of Care

Patient ratings of health care are an integral component of patient-centered care. In its definition of the essential dimensions of patient-centered care, the Institute of Medicine (now known as the National Academy of Medicine) includes shared decision making among clinicians, patients, and families; self-efficacy and self-management skills for patients; and the patient's experience of care.[66,67] Measurement of patient ratings is a complex concept that is related to perceived needs, expectations of care, and experience of care.[68-75] Patient ratings can cover the spectrum of patient engagement, from experience to shared decision making to self-management to full activation.

Clinicians' recognition of patient preferences and values can help health care professionals tailor treatments based on informed decisions that their patients might make based on those preferences. In fact, improving decision quality is one critically important step that the nation can take to improve the quality (processes and outcomes) of health care and thus enhance value for health care expenditures. For this reason, patients' ratings of their experiences with care not only provide information very salient to patients and families, but they also have considerable policy implications. Each safe practice in the updated NQF consensus report includes a section titled "Opportunities for Patient and Family Involvement."[76]

The three major types of patient health care ratings relate to evaluations of patient satisfaction, patient motivation and activation, and patient reports of their actual experiences. Patient satisfaction is a multidimensional construct that includes patient concerns about the disease and its treatment, issues of treatment affordability and financial burden for the patient, communication with health care providers, access to services, satisfaction with treatment explanations, and confidence in the physician.[77-83] Shikiar and Rentz proposed a three-level hierarchy of satisfaction: (1) satisfaction with health care delivery, including issues of accessibility, clinician-patient communication, and quality of facilities; (2) satisfaction with the treatment regimen, including medication, dietary and exercise recommendations, and similar elements of therapies; and (3) satisfaction with the medication itself, rather than the broader treatment.[73] Patient satisfaction has important implications for clinical decision making and enhancing the delivery of health care services; it is increasingly the focus of research and evaluation of medical treatments, services, and interventions.[84] It is an important indicator of future adherence to treatment.[72,85-90] Satisfaction has a long history of measurement, and numerous instruments are available.[70,75,91-99]

One potentially important predictor of health outcomes is patient activation, or the degree to which patients are motivated and have the relevant knowledge, skills, and confidence to make optimal health care decisions.[100-102] Hibbard and colleagues[102] developed a 13-item scale, the Patient Activation

Measure (PAM),[103,104] which demonstrated favorable psychometric properties in several cross-sectional and some longitudinal studies.[101] Although appreciation of the benefits of activated patients is increasing,[105] commensurate support is lacking to help patients become more activated with respect to their health care decision making.[104] Although research supports the claim that improvements in patient activation are associated with improvements in self-reported health behaviors,[101,105] additional research is necessary to better understand both these relationships and their relevance to actual behavior. Patient activation, as measured by the PAM or otherwise, may be a useful moderator or mediator of PROs that will in turn contribute to performance measurement.

An important contemporary focus is on measuring patient reports of their actual experiences with health care services.[106] Reports about care are often regarded as more specific, actionable, understandable, and objective than general ratings alone.[107,108] The Consumer Assessment of Healthcare Providers and Systems (CAHPS) program is a multiyear AHRQ initiative to support and promote the assessment of consumers' experiences with health care. The CAHPS program has two main goals: (1) to develop standardized patient questionnaires and (2) to generate tools and resources that produce understandable and usable comparative information for both consumers and health care providers. The CAHPS project has become a leading mechanism for the measurement of patient perspectives on health care access and quality.

Method and Mode of Administration, Data Collection, and Analysis

To accommodate the needs of patients with diverse linguistic, cultural, educational, and functional skills, clinicians and researchers require some flexibility in choosing appropriate methods and modes of questionnaire administration for PROMs.[109] Numerous issues complicate scoring and analyzing PROM response data. We first describe these methods issues (Table 3)—sources of reports, modes of administration, methods of administration, settings, and scoring—and then discuss barriers.

As with the earlier descriptions of core PRO categories such as health-related quality of life, we highlight in this section the critical issues for measurement methods—i.e., the advantages or drawbacks that users would most need to take into account. This information reflects standard measurement theory (classical or contemporary) and is based on decades of published research and theoretical papers and inputs from experts involved with projects such as PROMIS.

Table 3. PRO methods: characteristics, strengths, and limitations

Methodological Issue	Main Characteristics	Main Strengths	Main Limitations
Source of report			
Self	Person responds about himself or herself	• Expert on own experience	• Not always possible to assess directly, e.g., because of cognitive or communication deficits or age/ developmental level
Proxy	Person responds about someone else	• Useful when target of assessment is unable to respond • Can provide complementary information	• May not accurately represent subjective or other experiences

(continued)

Table 3. PRO methods: characteristics, strengths, and limitations *(continued)*

Methodological Issue	Main Characteristics	Main Strengths	Main Limitations
Mode of administration			
Self	Person self-administers PROM and records the responses	• Cost-effective • May yield more participant disclosure • Proceed at one's own pace	• Potential for missing data • Simple survey design (e.g., minimal skip patterns)
Interviewer	Interviewer reads questions aloud and records the responses	• More complex survey design (e.g., skip patterns) • Useful for respondents with reading, writing, or vision difficulties	• Interviewer costs • Potential for bias (interviewer bias, social desirability bias, acquiescent response sets)
Method of administration			
Paper-and-pencil	Patient self-administers PROM using paper and a writing utensil	• Cost-effective	• Prone to data entry errors • Data entry, scoring require more time • Less amenable to incorporation within EHR
Electronic	Patient self-administers PROM using computer- or telephone-based platform	• Interactive • Practical • Increased comfort for socially undesirable behaviors • Minimizes data entry errors • Immediate scoring, feedback • Amenable to incorporation within EHR	• Cost • Potential discomfort with technology • Accessibility • Measurement equivalence
Setting of administration			
Clinic	Patient completes PROMs when he or she arrives to clinic appointments	• Real-time assessment of outcomes • Feasibility with use of electronic methods of administration	• Impact on clinic flow • Interruptions resulting in missing data • Patient anxiety • Staff burden

(continued)

Table 3. PRO methods: characteristics, strengths, and limitations *(continued)*

Methodological Issue	Main Characteristics	Main Strengths	Main Limitations
Setting of administration *(continued)*			
Home	Patient completes PROMs at home before or between clinic visits	• Minimizes impact on clinic flow • Minimizes staff burden	• Accessibility • Health information privacy • Data security • Patient safety
Other	Patients complete PROMs at other types of settings (e.g., skilled nursing, rehabilitation)	• Feasibility with electronic methods of administration	• Cognitive capacity and potential need for proxy
Scoring			
Classical test theory	Raw scores	• Easy to implement and understand	• All items must be administered
Modern test theory	Probabilistic approach	• Enables CAT (tailored questions) • Shorter questionnaires with more precision	• Difficult to implement and understand

CAT, computer-assisted testing; EHR, electronic health record; PRO, patient-reported outcome; PROM, patient-reported outcome measure.

Source: Data are from *Data Collection Methods. Quality of Life and Pharmacoeconomics in Clinical Trials*[130] and *Psychological Aspects of Health-Related Quality of Life Measurement: Tests and Scales. Quality of Life and Pharmacoeconomics in Clinical Trials.*[131]

Modes and Methods Issues

Administering PRO instruments (PROMs) requires users to make decisions about three aspects of data collection (Figure 1):

- **Data source**—i.e., the source of the PRO (the patient or, in some cases, a proxy or other reporter)
- **Mode** by which information was recorded—i.e., self-administered or interviewer-administered
- **Method** used to capture the information (such as paper-and-pencil questionnaire or telephone- or computer-assisted technologies).

Each of these aspects is described below. These three aspects can be combined in various ways. For example, a patient might use the telephone to self-administer a PROM, or an interviewer might use a computer to read questions and record answers.

Figure 1. Types of respondent sources of data and modes and methods of administration

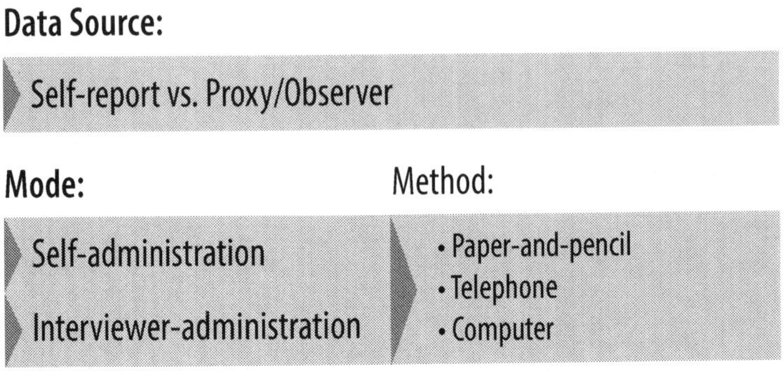

Data Source:

Self-report vs. Proxy/Observer

Mode: Method:

Self-administration   • Paper-and-pencil
                                     • Telephone
Interviewer-administration   • Computer

The patient's perspective is the focal point of PRO assessment. In some circumstances, directly obtaining this perspective may be difficult or impossible. In adults, cognitive and communications deficits and burden of disease, for example, can limit potential subjects' ability to complete PROMs.[110] This is especially likely to occur with the elderly and with people of any age who have severe disease or suffer from neurological disorders. Children's participation can be limited by these same factors plus issues specific to their age and developmental level.[110-112]

Failing to include these populations can result in potentially misleading interpretations of results. Thus, attempting to include them in PRO assessment efforts is crucial. Using all possible mechanisms for obtaining self-reports is a high priority, but accomplishing this may be out of the question for some populations.

Proxy Report as a Substitute for Self-Report

One way to include the greatest number of patients is to use proxy respondents to obtain PRO information for patients who are unable to respond. Using either significant others (e.g., parents, spouses or other family members, friends) or formal caregivers (physicians, nurses, aides, teachers) as proxies can provide many potential benefits. It not only allows inclusion of a broader and more representative range of patients in the entire measurement effort, but it can also help minimize missing data and increase the feasibility of longitudinal assessment.

The usefulness of proxy responses as *substitutes* for patient responses depends on the validity and reliability of proxy responses compared with those attributes for patient responses. When evaluating the quality of proxy responses, analysts usually compare proxy responses with patient responses. This is a reasonable approach, when proxy responses are being used to replace patient responses.

Agreement between the proxy and patient is typically assessed at either the subscale level, via the intraclass correlation coefficient (ICC), or the item level, by the kappa statistic, although other types of analyses have been advocated.[113] Patient and proxy responses are also often compared at the group level by comparing mean scores. Group comparisons help detect the magnitude and direction of any systematic bias that might be present.

Both the adult and pediatric literatures suggest that agreement between proxy and patient ratings is higher when rating observable functioning or HRQL dimensions such as physical and instrumental activities of daily living, physical health, and motor function. Agreement is typically lower for more subjective dimensions such as social functioning, pain, cognitive status or function, and psychological or emotional well-being.[112,114–118] Using continuous rather than dichotomous ratings improves agreement.[119] Extent of disagreement increases with increasing age of adolescents[120] and as the severity of patient illness, cognitive impairment, or disability rises.[121–124] Type of proxy (e.g., parent versus caregiver) and proxy characteristics such as age, education, and level of stress may also affect agreement.[125,126] In terms of direction of disagreement, proxies for adults tend to rate them as having more symptoms, functional difficulties, emotional distress, and negative quality of life; the main exception is pain, about which proxies tend to under-report.[114] Patterns of disagreement for child- versus proxy-reported outcomes are inconsistent.[127] Even when self- and proxy reports disagree for either children or adults, differences tend to be small.[127,128]

Proxy Report as a Complement to Self-Report

Proxy assessment may substitute for patient assessment where needed, but it may also complement it. Proxies can be asked to assess the patient as they think the patient would respond (i.e., proxy-patient perspective), or they can be asked to provide their own perspective on the patient's functioning or HRQL. This type of additional rating may be better described as either an external or "other" rating[129] for the sake of clarity. An important consideration is that the measure make clear which perspective is desired.[127]

The external (i.e., "other") perspective may provide particularly relevant information when the person is unable to provide any self-assessment, but it can be important even when the patient can give his or her own answers. In such cases, patient-other agreement may not necessarily be desirable. For example, patients in the earlier stages of dementia may be able to provide responses to PROMs but fail to recognize the extent of their impaired well-being and physical role functioning. In such cases, a next-of-kin caregiver such as a spouse could provide an external assessment that indicates that the patient has some degree of problems in functioning, such as getting the groceries from car to kitchen or being comfortable in a social setting. In these circumstances, external (proxy) respondents can clearly introduce clinically important information.

Mode: Self-Administration Versus Interviewer Administration

Self-administration of PROMs is neither expensive nor influenced by interviewer effects; for these reasons, this mode of administration has traditionally been preferred. However, self-administration is not feasible for some patient populations, such as those who may be too ill to self-administer a questionnaire. In these cases, interviewer administration is often required. Until recently, interviewer administration was also required for those with low literacy; however, new multimedia methods are now available to overcome this barrier.

Main Advantages and Disadvantages of Different Modes of Administration

Table 3 summarized the principal benefits and drawbacks of different modes of administration, based on authoritative sources.[130,131] Self-administered instruments are more cost-effective from a staffing perspective, and they may yield more patient disclosure, especially when collecting sensitive information.[132] Disadvantages include the potential for more missing data and the inability to clarify any misunderstandings in questions or response options.

By contrast, interviewer-administered instruments allow for probes and clarification, and they permit more complexity in survey design (e.g., the use of complicated skip patterns or open-ended questions). This mode is also useful for persons with reading, writing, or vision difficulties. Disadvantages include the costs required to hire, train, and supervise interviewers and the potential pressure on respondents to answer quickly, rather than letting them proceed at their own pace. The potential for interviewer bias cannot be overlooked.

It may arise from systematic differences from interviewer to interviewer or, occasionally, systematic errors on the part of many or even all interviewers.[133]

Additional Concerns About Sources of Bias

Other sources of bias for both administration modes include social desirability response set (the tendency to give a favorable picture of oneself) and acquiescent response set (the tendency to agree or disagree with statements regardless of their content).[134,135]

Legitimate concerns arise about the potential biasing effects of mode of administration on data quality and interpretation.[136] Overall, evidence supports high reliability for instruments administered with different modes, but response effects have varied and have not been consistently in the same direction.[121-124] For example, some studies have reported more favorable reports of well-being on self-administered questionnaires,[137] whereas others have found the opposite effect.[138-140] Still other studies reported mixed results[141] or found no important differences attributable to mode of administration after adjusting for other factors.[130,142,143] Fortunately, many types of error and bias can be overcome by appropriate selection and training of interviewers. Effects of different modes can also be evaluated with various psychometric and statistical techniques and models to determine the potential impact of response effects.[144-148]

Method of Administration

Advances in technology have changed the face of PROM assessment, increasing the number of administration options available. Multiple methods of self-administration currently exist, and the different methods may have different effects on the quality of the data.[136] Although diverse administration methods provide more options for researchers and clinicians, they require different skills and resources of people being asked to respond to the questionnaire. This means that the choice of method of administration may pose differing levels of respondent burden.[136]

Several factors may account for differences in data quality across methods of administration: impersonality of the method, cognitive burden on the respondent, ability to establish the legitimacy of the reasons for which patients or others are even being asked to complete a questionnaire, control over the questionnaires, and communication style.[136] Thus, when users are deciding on one (or more) appropriate methods of administration for a given PROM, they must give these factors due consideration.

Historically, paper-and-pencil administration served as the primary method of PROM assessment. Many PROMs were originally developed with the intention of paper-based administration, but they may be (and typically are) amenable to an electronic-based administration.[149] Paper-and-pencil remains a widely used PROM administration method, with its primary advantage being cost-effectiveness in situations in which users face few mailing and follow-up costs.

However, the paper-and-pencil method has disadvantages. For example, it may require that a person's responses be manually entered into a database for scoring purposes, raising the possibility of data entry errors that threaten the integrity of the results. Similarly, the need for manual data entry and scoring can be time-intensive. Although the availability of optical mark recognition and optical character recognition allow scanning of paper-and-pencil PROMs, this process still requires an extra step on the part of staff and may limit the acceptability of paper-and-pencil administration for purposes in which timely scoring and interpretation are important.

Advances in technology and the increasingly widespread availability of electronic resources have provided several alternatives to paper-and-pencil administration. Improved telephone technology has enabled the use of interactive voice response to administer PROMs. Interactive voice response involves a computer audio-recording of PROM questions administered via telephone to which people indicate their responses by selecting the appropriate key.[136,149]

In addition, computer-based administration methods have emerged as feasible alternatives to paper-and-pencil, such as web-based platforms, touchscreen computers, and multimedia platforms that can accommodate people with a range of literacy and computer skills (e.g., Talking Touchscreen/la Pantalla Parlanchina, audiovisual computer-assisted self-interviewing).[136,149-151] Newer mobile forms of technology such as tablet computers and smartphones also offer promise as methods of PROM administration.

Electronic administration methods have advantages that contribute to their increasingly widespread adoption. For example, because patients or respondents enter the data themselves, the opportunity for data entry errors is minimal compared with paper-and-pencil administration with separate data entry. These electronic methods also typically allow for immediate scoring and feedback, which enhances applications requiring timely results. Furthermore, electronic PROM administration has been shown to be practical, acceptable, and cost-effective.[60] Electronic methods may also provide people with increased comfort when responding to questions about socially undesirable behaviors.[152]

Nonetheless, these advantages must be considered in light of several important disadvantages. First, the cost of purchasing technology-based platforms may exceed that of traditional paper-and-pencil methods. Additionally, some patients may experience discomfort with technology or lack the skills necessary to navigate electronic administration methods. Moreover, reliance upon methods such as web-based platforms or smartphones raises questions about people's access to these technologies, if they are not provided in the relevant settings as part of clinical practice, quality improvement, or other assessment efforts.

The availability of multiple methods of PROM administration highlights the importance of measurement equivalence across methods.[149] Measurement equivalence is determined by comparing the psychometric properties of data obtained via paper-based administration and data collected through electronic administration.[149] It can be assessed via cognitive testing, usability testing, equivalence testing, or psychometric testing (or various combinations of these techniques).[149] A growing body of research documents the equivalence of electronic and paper-and-pencil administration of PROMs.[153–155] These findings support the viability of electronic PROM administration as an alternative to paper-and-pencil methods.

In addition to measurement equivalence, patient privacy is another concern that cuts across both paper-and-pencil and electronic administration methods, albeit in differing ways. For paper-based PROMs, physical transfer of the PROM from patient to provider, as well as the physical existence of the completed PROM, may pose risks to the privacy and confidentiality of patients' responses. Privacy also emerges as a concern about electronic methods, given potential security breaches related to transfer of data, computer errors, or unauthorized access to patient-reported data. These threats underscore the need for reliable and secure electronic platforms to protect patients' privacy in the context of PROM assessment.

Patient-Reported Outcome Measures in the Clinical Setting

Collecting PRO data as part of clinical care has become common.[2,156–158] Facilitating introduction of these PROMs into clinical practice and decision making promises many benefits. Advocates for using PROMs in clinical care propose that the results assist clinical providers in managing their patients' care,[159] enhance the efficiency of clinical practice,[155,160] improve patient-provider communication,[155,160-162] identify patient needs in a timely manner,[155, 163] and facilitate patient-centered care.[155] Other findings, however, suggest regional variation in perceived health and no positive effect of feedback via PROMs on care, even when combined with guideline-recommended interventions.[164-166] As PROMs are used more in clinical practice, some methodological issues pertaining to the settings in which they are administered merit consideration.

A growing number of studies have investigated the use of PROMs in the clinic setting.[155,160,162,163,167-170] When selecting PROMs for administration in clinical practice, users need to consider the efficiency of PROM administration, scoring, and interpretation. These factors are especially important because of the time-sensitive nature of the clinic workflow.[155,167] In addition, acceptability of both the PROM and the data collection process for both patients and clinic staff is essential.[155,167,171]

Historically, several barriers have impeded widespread implementation of PRO data collection in clinical settings of all sorts, but especially for smaller or private practices. Many drawbacks are associated with paper-and-pencil administration of PROMs. One such barrier involves concerns about the potential disruption to the clinical workflow if patients are asked to complete PROMs.[159] In addition, staff burden and clinician disengagement may hamper obtaining PRO data in clinical settings.[159]

Fortunately, technology advances, and the increased opportunities for methods of PROM administration that they afford, may help to overcome some barriers to PRO data collection in clinical practices and settings.[167] For example, research supports the feasibility of using tablet computers[155,163] and touchscreen computers for these purposes.[150,151,162,167,168] Employing computers to administer PROMs may streamline and expedite the process and minimize staff burden and impact on clinic flow.

Conversely, concerns arise regarding the impact of clinic flow on the integrity of data collection, given the potential for patients to be interrupted while completing PROMs, which could potentially result in missing data.[159] Another potential barrier involves the possibility that patients may experience anxiety in completing PROMs in the clinical settings before their appointments.[159] Similarly, a possible lack of privacy when completing PROMs in waiting rooms or similar circumstances poses another potential obstacle to adequate PROM administration. Many of these concerns can be addressed by incorporating PROMs into the clinical workflow. This may also enhance completion rates. Both patients and providers will then be more likely to see this effort as integral to patient care.

Completing PROMs from home before or between medical appointments has been proposed as one strategy to overcoming the problems outlined above.[159,172,173] Both web-based PROM administration and interactive voice response constitute possible methods for at-home PRO data collection.[151,161,162] Although the home may serve as a feasible alternative to the clinical practice setting for various reasons, those considering implementing home-based PRO data collection need to consider several factors.[159,172] First, for patients to be able to complete PROMs at home, they must have access to the type of technology by which the PROM is administered (e.g., Internet). Second, patients must find completing PROMs at home acceptable. Third, users should have a plan in place to address situations in which home-based PROM responses suggest critical or acute problems. This may pose a logistical challenge in comparison with PROMs completed in-clinic, where medical providers and access to intervention are readily available.

As with any setting, health information privacy is paramount; therefore, one barrier to home-based PROMs is the availability of secure data collection platforms.[159,174] Finally, an especially difficult issue may be clinician acceptability of home-based PRO data collection. The problems include reimbursement for clinicians' time using a website to address outcomes that patients report, rather than meeting directly with patients to discuss questions or problems that their patients raise through answers to the PROMs.[159,174]

Implementing PRO data collection in other settings, such as rehabilitation or skilled nursing facilities, may also yield valuable clinical information and guide interventions. Less research has addressed the issues in administering PROMs in these settings. However, handheld technology may offer a means of facilitating collection of PRO data in the rehabilitation setting following orthopedic surgery.[175]

Apart from technology per se, other issues in such facilities include the varying level of patients' acuity status and levels of cognitive capacity to complete PROMs. In these cases, users may need to consider whether using proxy reports may be beneficial. In any case, the potential strengths and weaknesses of different modes and methods of administration still need to be taken into account.

Scoring: Classical Test Theory Versus Modern Test Theory

Many PROMs involve the measurement of *latent* (not directly observable) variables; examples might include symptoms (not signs) of gastrointestinal disease or pain. The only way to estimate a person's level on a particular attribute is by asking questions that represent the attribute in question. Most PROMs comprise multiple items that are aggregated in some way to produce an overall score. The most common multi-item instruments are designed to reflect a single underlying construct. The item responses either are caused by or are manifestations of the underlying latent attribute, and the items are expected to correlate with one another.[176–179]

In some other kinds of multi-item measures, the items may cluster together but would not be expected to correlate. A common example of this latter measure is a comorbidity index comprising various health conditions, e.g., diabetes, asthma, and heart disease. Another example might be a measure of access to care consisting of problems with paying for care, having a regular provider, ease of transportation to care, and ease of making an appointment. Although such items would not necessarily be correlated, together they might form an adequate measure of access. The discussion on scoring below refers to the former type of instrument reflecting underlying constructs with items expected to correlate with one another.

Scoring is based on classical test theory (raw scores) or modern test theory (item response theory [IRT]).[180–189] Multiple items are preferred because a response to a single item provides only limited information to distinguish among individuals.[190] In addition, measurement error (the difference between the true score and the observed score) tends to average out when responses to individual items are summed to obtain a total score.[190–192]

Classical test theory estimates the level of an attribute as the sum, perhaps weighted, of responses to individual items, i.e., as a linear combination.[13,190,193–196] This approach requires *all* items on a particular PROM to be used in every situation for it to be considered valid. Hence, the instrument is *test-dependent*.[194,196–198]

IRT, by contrast, enables *test-free* measurement; i.e., the latent trait can be estimated using different items as long as their locations (difficulty levels) have been calibrated on the same scale as the patients' ability levels.[13,190,196–201] IRT allows computer-adaptive testing (CAT) in which the number, order, and content of the questions are tailored to the individual patient. This approach has two distinct advantages: (1) questionnaires can be shorter, and (2) the scale scores can be estimated more precisely for any given test length. This also means that different patients do not need to complete the same set of items in every situation.[13]

Using IRT poses nontrivial challenges, however. Understanding the assumptions and the psychometric jargon—e.g., "calibration," "difficulty levels"—is not easy. The methodology and software are complex. IRT is also not appropriate for causal variables and complex latent traits.[13,196,197,202] Overall, however, IRT offers a very convenient and efficient framework for PRO measurement, and it is becoming increasingly well understood and easier to adopt.

Linking or Cross-Talk Between Different Measures of the Same Construct

A common problem when using an array of health-related outcomes for diverse patient populations and subgroups is establishing the comparability of scales or units on which the outcomes are reported.[203,204] Typically the metric has been emphasized more than the measure. *Equating* is a technique to convert the system of units of one measure to that of another. Analysts have successfully used this process of deriving equivalent scores in educational testing to compare test scores obtained from parallel or alternate forms that measure the same characteristic with or without having common anchor items.

Theoretically (and in practice when certain conditions are met), different age-specific measures could be linked, thus placing child, adult, and geriatric estimates on a common metric. For example, the many items that constitute a condition-specific (e.g., cancer) quality of life scale could be incorporated into a single shared bank and linked through a common-anchor design.[203] The methods of establishing comparable scores—often called *linking*—vary substantially depending on the definition of comparability. For that reason, standardization is critical in comparing PROMs across studies. Two measures may be considered linked if they produce scores that match the first two moments of their distributions (i.e., mean and standard deviation for a specific group of examinees or two randomly equivalent groups). Another definition may involve matching scores with equal percentile ranks based on a single sample of examinees or random samples drawn from the same population.

Addressing Barriers to Patient-Reported Outcomes Measurement

Users need to address yet other barriers to PRO measurement. These include administering PROMs in vulnerable populations; literacy, health literacy, and numeracy; language and cultural differences; differences in functional abilities; response shift; use of different methods and modes of administration; and the impact of nonresponders to items and questionnaires. In discussing these issues below, we also note best practices and recommendations for addressing them.

Vulnerable Populations

Recognition is growing that some population subgroups are particularly vulnerable to receiving suboptimal health care and to failing to achieve health outcomes equivalent to those experienced by the general population.[205–207] Vulnerability is multifaceted. It can arise from age, race, ethnicity, or sex (or gender); health, functional, or developmental status; financial circumstances (income, health insurance); place of residence; or ability to communicate effectively.[205] Moreover, many of these factors are synergistic, so that vulnerability has many sources that present a complicated picture for persons in these groups. This definition encompasses populations who are vulnerable because of a chronic or terminal illness or disability and those with literacy or language difficulties.[150,206] It also includes people residing in areas with health professional shortages.[168]

Administration of PROMs is usually performed with paper-and-pencil instruments, and multilingual versions of questionnaires are often not available. Interviewer administration is labor-intensive and cost-prohibitive in most health care settings. Therefore, patients with low literacy, those with certain functional limitations, and those who do not speak English are typically excluded, either explicitly or implicitly, from any outcome evaluation in a clinical practice setting in which patient-reported data are collected on forms.

As PROs continue to play a greater role in medical decision making and evaluation of the quality of health care, sensitive and efficient methods of measuring those outcomes among underserved populations must be developed and validated. Minority status, language preference, and literacy level may be critical variables in differentiating those who receive and respond well to treatment from those who do not. These patients may experience different health outcomes because of disparities in care or barriers to care.

Outcome measurement in these patients may provide new insight into disease or treatment problems that may have gone undetected simply because many studies have not been able to accommodate the special needs of such patients.[206,208]

Literacy

Low literacy is a widespread but neglected problem in the United States. The 1992 National Adult Literacy Survey (NALS)[209] and the 2003 National Assessment of Adult Literacy (NAAL)[210] measured three kinds of English language literacy tasks that adults encounter in daily life (prose literacy, document literacy, quantitative literacy). Almost half of the adult population experiences difficulty in using reading, speaking, writing, and computational skills in everyday life situations. An additional seven million adults in the US population were estimated to be nonliterate in English. Generally speaking, *health* literacy problems complicate matters of both health care delivery and PRO measurement.[211,212]

Health literacy is "the degree to which individuals have the capacity to obtain, process, and understand basic health information and services needed to make appropriate health decisions."[213] This involves using a range of skills (e.g., reading, listening, speaking, writing, numeracy) to function effectively in the health care environment and act appropriately on health care information.[214, 215] Limited health literacy is widespread[214,216] and is associated with medication errors, increased health care costs, hospitalizations, increased mortality, decreased self-efficacy, and inadequate knowledge and self-care for chronic health conditions.[211,214,217–219] Health literacy may be more limiting than functional literacy because of the unfamiliar context and vocabulary of the health care system.[212,214,220]

Contributing to poor understanding of the importance of literacy skills is the fact that low literacy is often underreported. The NALS reported that 66 percent to 75 percent of adults in the lowest reading level and 93 percent to 97 percent in the second-lowest reading level described themselves as being able to read or write English "well" or "very well."[209] In addition, low-literacy individuals are frequently ashamed of their reading difficulties and try to hide the problem, even from their families.[221,222] Lack of recognition and denial of reading problems create a barrier to health care. Some low-literacy patients have acknowledged avoiding medical care because they are ashamed of their reading difficulties.[221,222] In addition, because everyday life may place only moderate reading demands on people, individuals may not even be aware of their reading problems until a literacy-challenging event occurs (e.g., reviewing treatment options, reading a consent document, completing health assessment forms).[221,222]

A reader's comprehension of text depends on the purpose for reading, the ability of the reader, and the text that is being read. Two important factors in the readability of text are word familiarity and sentence length.[223] Unfamiliar words are difficult when first encountered. Long sentences are likely to contain more phrases or clauses. Although longer sentences may communicate more information and more ideas, they are more difficult for readers to manage than more, but shorter, sentences that convey the same information. Moreover, longer sentences may also require the reader to retain more information in short-term memory.[224-227]

Addressing health literacy is now recognized as critical to delivering person-centered health care.[228] It is an important component of providing quality health care to diverse populations, and it will be incorporated into the National Standards for Culturally and Linguistically Appropriate Services.[229] For example, translating highly technical medical and legal language into easily understood language is challenging, whether into English or another language. Health literacy practices are also included in the National Quality Forum 2010 updated set of safe practices.[76] A recent discussion paper summarized 10 attributes that exemplify a "health literate health care organization."[228] These attributes cover practical strategies across all aspects of health care, from leadership planning and evaluation, to workforce training, to clear communication practices for patients.

Language and Culture

The availability of multiple language versions of PROMs has enabled users to administer them relatively routinely in diverse research and practice settings. For various purposes, doing analyses on data that have been pooled across all patients is desirable. Yet concern is often voiced about combining data from different cultures or languages.[10] In some research and practice-based initiatives, evaluating cross-cultural differences in PROMs is of interest. In all these applications, researchers must use unbiased questionnaires that can detect important differences among patients.[206,230,231]

Possible cultural differences in interpreting questions and in response styles may limit data pooling or may constrain comparisons across members of different cultural groups.[232-234] Similarly, poor quality translations can produce noncomparable language versions of PROMs.[233,235,236] For a questionnaire to be suitable for use as an unbiased measure of a PRO, items in the questionnaire must perform similarly across different groups (i.e., they must be cross-culturally or cross-linguistically equivalent).[231,237-248] Without assurances that the PROM is culturally and linguistically "fair," detected treatment differences caused by items that function differently across groups could incorrectly be interpreted to reflect real treatment differences. Similarly, differences in questionnaire performance may mask true treatment differences, especially when language or cultural groups are not balanced across the populations, practices, or settings to be compared.

Functional Abilities

Ideally, PROMs that are intended to be used in performance measurement applications can be completed by all patients in the target populations. Otherwise, if a significant proportion of the population is left out, the remaining individuals being assessed may be unrepresentative of the whole practice or setting. This problem can (and probably will) compromise the validity of the performance measure.

Functional limitations associated with disability are one type of potential barrier to PRO assessment that could affect PRO use in performance measurement. The prevalence of disability, defined as specific functional or sensory limitations, is estimated at 47.5 million Americans, or 22 percent of the US population.[249] People with a disability are more likely to develop health conditions and be consumers of health care than those with no disabilities of these types. Thus, they are an important group to include when evaluating health care, but one that is frequently not included in such clinical, quality improvement, or simulation initiatives.[250,251]

Common disabilities that can affect PROM assessment include problems with vision (e.g., decreased visual acuity, color-blindness), hearing, motor skills (e.g., upper extremity limitations), and cognitive deficits (e.g., impaired comprehension, reading). Fortunately, to address many of these barriers, those administering such measures have a variety of techniques: choosing appropriate methods and modes of data collection, enabling use of assistive devices and technology, and using principles of universal design when developing instruments.[201-202]

Universal design refers to designing products and environments in such a way that all people can use them, to the greatest extent possible, without adaptation or specialization.[252,253] A well-known example of universal design is the use of curb cuts. Initially intended to facilitate the use of wheelchairs, curb cuts have also benefited bicycle riders and people pushing children in strollers, among others. An exhaustive examination of how to apply the principles of universal design to PROM assessment is beyond the scope of this paper, and those developing or modifying measures according to the principles of universal design are encouraged to consult with relevant experts. Also, if developers are creating an instrument based on information technologies, using the standards in Section 508 of the Rehabilitation Act Amendments of 1998 can maximize flexibility.[254] Although we cannot list all potential ways to address functional limitations, we identify below some common ways to do so. Harniss and colleagues describe how PROMIS is taking a systematic approach to enhancing accessibility.[255]

In general, providing multiple means of understanding and responding to measures is important. These include visual, voiced, and tactile mechanisms. The specific means may differ depending on the method and mode of administration.

For instance, for people with impaired vision, one might consider using in-person or telephone interviews (advantages and disadvantages discussed in an earlier section), an interative voice response system, Braille responses for Braille users, or touchscreen with tactile or audio cues. Information technology-based systems should accommodate assistive devices such as screen readers and screen-enlargement software. For patients with hearing impairments, options include providing visual presentation of words or images, using TTY (text telephones) or a video relay service, and allowing the user to adjust the sound level. For persons with motor limitations, response modes that are easier to manipulate (track ball) or are nonmotoric (e.g., using voice recognition software) can be helpful. For those with certain types of cognitive deficits (e.g., limited reading comprehension), the methods to address literacy described earlier should be considered. However, if cognitive deficits are severe, a proxy respondent may be more appropriate.

Allowing for multiple response modes or methods may lead to measurement error. In a later section, we discuss the potential impact of different methods and modes on response rate, reliability, and validity. The risk of introducing measurement error seems outweighed by the risk of excluding a significant segment of the population.

Response Shift, Adaptation, and Other Challenges to Detecting True Change

The ability to detect true change over time in PROMs poses another barrier to the integrity of valid PRO assessment. Often, detecting true change is associated with the phenomenon of *response shift*. This has been defined as "a change in the meaning of one's self-evaluation of a target construct as a result of: (a) a change in the respondent's internal standards of measurement (i.e., scale recalibration); (b) a change in the respondent's values (i.e., the importance of component domains constituting the target construct); or (c) a redefinition of the target construct (i.e., reconceptualization)."[256,p.1532] A change in perspective over time may result in patients' attending to PROMs in a systematically different way from one time point to another.[257]

Response shift serves as a barrier to PRO assessment for several important reasons. For example, it threatens longitudinal PRO assessment validity, reliability, and responsiveness.[257–260] Response shift can complicate the interpretation of PROM scores; a change in a PROM may occur because of response shift, an effect of treatment, or both.[261]

Monitoring for response shift can aid PROM users in interpreting longitudinal PRO data.[259] Several strategies have been proposed to identify response shift, although each has limitations. The "then test" compares an actual pre-test rating and a retrospective pre-test rating to assess for shift, but it is less robust than other methods of detecting response shift[257] and it is confounded with recall bias.[260] Structural equation modeling has also been proposed as a way to identify response shift, but it is sensitive only if most of the sample is likely to make response shifts.[262] Finally, growth modeling creates a predictive growth curve model to investigate patterns in discrepancies between expected and observed scores, thus assessing response shift at the individual level.[263] Although growth modeling enables users to detect both the timing and shape of response shift,[259] it cannot differentiate between random error and response shift.[260]

Implications of the Different Methods and Modes for Response Rate, Reliability, and Validity

Implementing Data Collection Methods

Users of PROMs must make a variety of decisions about the data collection method and the implications of those decisions on costs and errors in surveys.[132] Two basic issues underlie these decisions: What is the most appropriate method to choose for a particular question, and What is the impact of a particular method on survey errors and costs?

Methods differ along a variety of dimensions.[132] These include, although are not limited to, the degree of interviewer involvement and the level of interaction with the respondent. Channels of communication (sight, sound, touch) may prompt different issues of comprehension, memory stimulation, social influence affecting judgment, and response hurdles. Finally, the degree of technology use is a major consideration.

Using Different Method or Mode Than the One Originally Validated

Considering the implications of using a different method or mode than the one on which the PROM was originally validated is also important. Many existing PROMs were initially validated in paper-and-pencil form. However, potential differences exist between paper-and-pencil and electronic-based PROM administration, ranging from differences in how items and responses are presented (e.g., items presented one at a time, size of text) to differences in participant comfort level in responding (e.g., ability to interact with electronic-based platforms).[153]

As noted earlier, a growing body of research suggests measurement equivalence between paper- and computer-administered PROMs.[153,264] However, the effect of a particular data collection method on a particular source of error may depend on the specific combination of methods used.[132] Thus, as new methods are developed, studies comparing them with the methods they may replace must be done.

In framing expectations about the likely effect of a particular approach, developers need to invoke theories about that approach. Theory is informed by past mode-effects literature and by an understanding of the features or elements of a particular design.[132] Similarly, mode choices involve trade-offs and compromises. Therefore, the choice of a particular approach must be made within the context of the particular objectives of the survey and the resources available.[132]

Using Multiple Methods and Modes

The implications of using multiple methods and modes also warrant consideration. One might choose to blend methods for one or more reasons: cost reduction, faster data collection, optimization of response rates.[132] When combining methods or modes (or both), users must ensure that they can disentangle any effects of the method or mode from other population characteristics. This is especially true when respondents choose which method or mode they prefer or when access issues determine the choice of method or mode.[132] As in the case of using a different method or mode than the one in which the PROM was originally validated, instruments and procedures should be designed with an eye to ensuring equivalence across both methods and modes.[265]

Accounting for the Impact of Nonresponders

Difficulties with data collection and questionnaire completion are major barriers to the successful implementation of PRO assessment. The principal problem is that missing data can introduce bias in analyses, findings, and conclusions or recommendations.[13] The choice of mode and method of questionnaire administration can affect nonresponse rates and nonresponse bias.[132] In addition, often the timing of the assessment can be very important, e.g., just before or just after surgery.

Missing data may be classified as either item nonresponse (one or more missing items within a questionnaire) or unit nonresponse (the whole questionnaire is missing for a patient). Evaluating the amount of, reasons for, and patterns of missing data is important.[266-269] Some common strategies to evaluate nonresponse bias include

- conducting an abbreviated follow-up survey with initial nonrespondents[132]

- comparing characteristics of respondents and nonrespondents[270,271]

- comparing respondent data with comparable information from other sources[272]

- comparing on-time vs. late respondents.[273]

When dealing with missing data, analysts can use various statistical methods of adjustment. For item nonresponse in multi-item scales, several useful techniques tend to yield unbiased estimates of scores: simple mean imputation, regression imputation, and IRT models. For both item and unit nonresponse, it is important to determine whether missing data are considered to be missing completely at random (MCAR), missing at random (MAR), or missing not at random (MNAR).[266,267] For unit nonresponse, users can implement a range of statistical techniques, depending on the reason for missing data.[274-278]

Selection of Patient-Level PROMs

Patient-Centered Outcomes Research

An essential aspect of patient-centered outcomes research (PCOR) is the integration of patient perspectives and experiences with clinical and biological data collected from the patient to evaluate the safety and efficacy of an intervention. Such integration recognizes that although traditional clinical endpoints such as laboratory values or survival are still very important, we also need to look at how disease and treatment affects patients' health-related quality of life (HRQL). For such HRQL endpoints, in most cases, the patients are the best source for reporting what they are experiencing. The challenge is how best to capture patient data in a way that maximizes our ability to inform decision making in the research, health care delivery, and policy settings.

Access to psychometrically sound and decision-relevant PROMs will allow clinicians, investigators, administrators, and others to collect empirical evidence on the differential benefits and harms of a health-related intervention.[279-282] Those obtaining such information can then disseminate findings to patients, clinicians and health care professionals, payers or insurers, and policy makers. Doing so may provide a richer perspective on the net impact of interventions on patients' lives using endpoints that are meaningful to the patients.[283]

Increasingly, longitudinal observational and experimental studies have included PROMs. To optimize decision making in clinical care, users must assess these PROMs in a standardized way, using questionnaires that demonstrate specific measurement properties.[279,282,284-287] Our group recently identified minimum standards for the design or selection of a PROM for use in PCOR activities.[288] Central to this work was understanding which attributes would make a PROM appropriate or inappropriate for such purposes. We identified these standards through two complementary approaches. The first was to conduct an extensive review of the literature including both published and unpublished guidance documents. The second was to assemble a group of international experts in PROMs and PCOR efforts to seek consensus on the minimum standards.[288]

Attributes of PROMs

Many documents summarize attributes of a good HRQL measure. They include (an illustrative list) guidance documents from the FDA;[289–292] the 2002 Medical Outcomes Trust guidelines on attributes of a good HRQL measure;[293] the extensive, international expert-driven recommendations from COSMIN (COnsensus-based Standards for the selection of health Measurement INstruments);[285,294–298] the EORTC (European Organization for Research and Treatment of Cancer) guidelines for developing questionnaires;[299] the Functional Assessment of Chronic Illness Therapy (FACIT) approach;[36] the International Society for Pharmacoeconomics and Outcomes Research (ISPOR) task force recommendation documents;[149,241,300,301] and several others.[245,284,302–304] Since 2010, ISOQOL (the International Society of Quality of Life) has completed two important guidance documents on use of PROMs in comparative effectiveness research and on integrating PROMs in health care delivery settings.[284,305] Finally, the NIH PROMIS network released a standards document in 2012 that is useful for informing the minimal and optimal standards for designing PROMs.[306]

Table 4 presents long-established criteria to consider in selecting PROMs for research, quality improvement activities, and now performance measurement. It specifies issues that PROM users need to consider when contemplating incorporating PROMs into performance measures and offers some best practices for evaluating PROMs in this context.

The eight primary criteria are the following: (1) conceptual or measurement model; (2) reliability and its subparts (e.g., internal consistency reliability); (3) validity and its subparts (e.g., content validity); (4) how scores are interpreted; (5) burden placed on respondents; (6) alternative modes and methods of administration; (7) cultural and language adaptations; and (8) use of electronic health records (EHRs). The table does not specify key issues and best practices for reliability or validity; that information is given only for the subcriteria. We illustrate these points with selected information pertaining to the Western Ontario and McMaster Universities Osteoarthritis Index (WOMAC).[307]

Table 4. Primary criteria for evaluating and selecting patient-reported outcome measures (PROMs) for use in performance measurement

Criteria and Subcriteria for Evaluating PROMs	Specific Issues to Address for Performance Measures and Best Practices in Assessing Candidate PROMs	Example: The Western Ontario and McMaster Universities Osteoarthritis Index (WOMAC)[307] for Use in Hip Arthroplasty
1. Conceptual and Measurement Model		
• Documentation should define and describe the concept(s) included and the intended population(s) for use. • Documentation should explain how the concept(s) are organized into a measurement framework, including evidence for the dimensionality of the measure, how items relate to each measured concept, and the relationships among concepts.	• Target PRO concept should be a high priority for the health care system and patients. • Patient engagement should define what an important concept to patients is. • Target PRO concept must be actionable in response to the health care intervention.	• Patient input was used to evaluate the dimensionality and the importance of concepts to be measured.[308] • Evidence suggests that some items measure the theoretically different concepts of physical function and pain load together on the same factor.[309]
2. Reliability		
Documentation should specify the degree to which an instrument is free from random error.	Adequate levels of reliability are prerequisites for determining the potential use of any PROM.	See 2a and 2b for WOMAC examples.
2a. Internal consistency (multi-item scales)		
Documentation should be provided about the reliability of a multi-item scale each time it is used; this should include the sample size, the number of items, and the specific reliability coefficient used.	Classical test theory (CTT) typically relies on the following values: • Reliability estimate ≥ 0.70 for group-level scores • Reliability estimate ≥ 0.90 for individual-level scores Item response theory (IRT) typically uses the following: • Item information curves that demonstrate precision[189] • A formula that can be applied to estimate CTT reliability.	Cronbach's alphas for the three subscales (pain, stiffness, and physical function) range from 0.86 to 0.98.[310–312]

(continued)

Table 4. Primary criteria for evaluating and selecting patient-reported outcome measures (PROMs) for use in performance measurement *(continued)*

Criteria and Subcriteria for Evaluating PROMs	Specific Issues to Address for Performance Measures and Best Practices in Assessing Candidate PROMs	Example: The Western Ontario and McMaster Universities Osteoarthritis Index (WOMAC)[307] for Use in Hip Arthroplasty
2. Reliability *(continued)*		
2b. Reproducibility (stability over time)		
Documentation should be provided about the specific reproducibility estimate used and the justification for the length of time between assessments.	For evaluating trends or changes over time, an adequate level of reproducibility is a prerequisite for determining the potential use of any PROM.	Test-retest reliability has been adequate for the pain and physical function subscales, but less adequate for the stiffness subscale.[312]
3. Validity		
Documentation should explain the degree to which the instrument reflects what it is supposed to measure.	• A limited number of PROMs have been validated for performance measurement. • PROMs should include questions that are patient-centered.	See 3a, 3b, and 3c for WOMAC examples.
3a. Content Validity		
Documentation should explain the extent to which a measure samples a representative range of the content that it is supposed to cover, whether for the populations, settings, or other elements of the measurement task.	A PROM should have evidence supporting its content validity, including evidence that patients or experts (or both) consider the content of the PROM relevant and comprehensive for the concept, population, and aim of the measurement application. Meeting this criterion may entail: • documenting the qualitative or quantitative methods (or both) used to solicit and confirm attributes (i.e., concepts measured by the items) of the PROM relevant to the measurement application. • documenting the characteristics of participants included in the evaluation (e.g., race/ethnicity, culture, age, socioeconomic status, literacy). • documenting sources from which items were derived, modified, and prioritized during the PROM development process. • giving an adequate justification for the recall period for the measurement application.	Development involved expert clinician input, survey input from patients,[308] and a review of existing measures.

(continued)

Table 4. Primary criteria for evaluating and selecting patient-reported outcome measures (PROMs) for use in performance measurement *(continued)*

Criteria and Subcriteria for Evaluating PROMs	Specific Issues to Address for Performance Measures and Best Practices in Assessing Candidate PROMs	Example: The Western Ontario and McMaster Universities Osteoarthritis Index (WOMAC)[307] for Use in Hip Arthroplasty
3. Validity *(continued)*		
3b. Construct and Criterion-Related Validity		
Documentation should explain how the PROM meets standard requirements for these two types of validity, giving appropriate evidence (empirical findings).	A PROM should have evidence that • supports predefined hypotheses about the expected associations among measures that are similar to or dissimilar from the measured PRO. • supports predefined hypotheses of the expected differences in scores between or among "known" groups. • shows the extent to which scores of the instrument are related to a criterion measure.	• Patient ratings of satisfaction with arthroplasty were correlated with WOMAC scores in the expected direction.[30,313,314] • Scores differentiated between patients with better versus worse outcomes after knee arthroplasty[30] and between patients with less versus more severe osteoarthritis.[315]
3c. Responsiveness		
For longitudinal initiatives or applications, documentation should explain how the PROM can detect change over time and change in response to an intervention (i.e., empirical findings of changes in scores consistent with predefined hypotheses regarding changes in the target population).	• If a PROM has cross-sectional data that provide sufficient evidence in regard to the reliability (internal consistency), content validity, and construct validity but has no data yet on responsiveness over time (i.e., ability of a PROM to detect changes in the construct being measured over time), users need to consider carefully whether such a measure is likely to provide valid data over time in a longitudinal study, especially if no other PROM is available. • Emphasizing responsiveness is important because of the expectation that care will have consequences. If action is to be taken, then demonstrating responsiveness is important. • PROMs must be sensitive to detect change in response to the specific health care intervention.	Responsiveness and ability to detect change in response to clinical intervention are both adequate.[316]

(continued)

Table 4. Primary criteria for evaluating and selecting patient-reported outcome measures (PROMs) for use in performance measurement *(continued)*

Criteria and Subcriteria for Evaluating PROMs	Specific Issues to Address for Performance Measures and Best Practices in Assessing Candidate PROMs	Example: The Western Ontario and McMaster Universities Osteoarthritis Index (WOMAC)[307] for Use in Hip Arthroplasty
4. Interpretability of Scores		
Documentation should support and assist users in interpreting scores from the PRO measure, including: • What low and high scores represent for the measured concept • Representative mean(s) and standard deviation(s) in the reference population • Guidance on the minimally important difference in scores between groups or over time (or both) that can be considered meaningful from patient and clinical perspectives.	• If different PROMs are used, establishing a link or crosswalk between them is important. • Because the criteria for assessing clinically important change in individuals do not directly translate to evaluating clinically important group differences,[317] a useful strategy is to calculate the proportion of patients who experience a clinically significant change.[280,317]	• Population-based, age- and sex- (or gender-) normative values are available.[318] • Minimal clinically important improvement values are available.[319] • Instrument can be translated into a utility score for use in economic and accountability evaluations.[320]
5. Burden		
Documentation should specify the time, effort, and other demands on both the respondent and the administrator.	• In a busy clinic setting, PRO assessment should be as brief as possible, and reporting should be done in real time. • Patient engagement should inform what constitutes "burden."	• Short form is available.[321] • Average time to complete mobile phone WOMAC is 4.8 minutes.[322]
6. Alternative Modes and Methods of Administration		
Documentation should specify participant and administration burden and information about comparability across the modes and methods of administration.	Using multiple modes and methods can be helpful for diverse populations. However, evidence regarding their equivalence is needed.	Validated mobile telephone- and touchscreen-based platforms are available.[323,324]

(continued)

Table 4. Primary criteria for evaluating and selecting patient-reported outcome measures (PROMs) for use in performance measurement *(continued)*

Criteria and Subcriteria for Evaluating PROMs	Specific Issues to Address for Performance Measures and Best Practices in Assessing Candidate PROMs	Example: The Western Ontario and McMaster Universities Osteoarthritis Index (WOMAC)[307] for Use in Hip Arthroplasty
7. Cultural and Language Adaptations		
Documentation should describe methods to evaluate cultural and linguistic equivalence.	The mode, method, and question wording must yield equivalent estimates of PRO measures.	Instrument is available in more than 65 languages.[325]
8. Electronic Health Records		
Documentation should describe key considerations for incorporation into electronic health records.	Critical features include: • Interoperability • Automated, real-time measurement and reporting • Sophisticated analytic capacities.	Electronic data capture may allow for integration within electronic health records.[322]

Note: This table is adapted from recommendations in a report from the Scientific Advisory Committee of the Medical Outcomes Trust[293] and a report submitted to the Methodology Committee of the Patient Centered Outcomes Research Institute.[288] We adapted the key points from these sources to enhance relevance to PRO selection for performance measurement.

Important Differences in PROM Attributes

Selecting PROMs for use in performance measurement and related activities such as quality improvement programs raises the question of what are the key differences, if any, when selecting PROMs for research purposes rather than these other nonresearch purposes. Generally speaking, the factors to consider when selecting PROMs for performance measurement and quality improvement activities are more similar than different. Thus, we focus here more on the differences that users will need to take into account.

Instrument Length

One key difference involves the length of the PROM. Longer questionnaires may be better tolerated in the context of research than in clinical practice settings; thus, to facilitate widespread adoption, PROMs for performance measurement should be short surveys. Addressing the need for shorter PROMs may, however, compromise other important measurement characteristics, such as reliability (i.e., precision and reproducibility).

Implications of PRO Data for Action

Another key difference in factors to consider when selecting PROMs for clinical practice quality improvement, or performance measurement and accountability efforts, is the implications or consequences of the PRO data. Specifically, using PROMs for these purposes carries the expectation that important consequences will arise in terms of accountability for health care professionals, health care systems and plans, and clinical settings. Therefore, the stakes of PROMs are higher in the performance measurement context than in research applications.

The problem lies, in part, in the constraints to the quality of the measurement level arising from factors unique to performance measurement. These can include instrument length or representativeness of the patient or consumer populations surveyed. These considerations highlight the importance of emphasizing responsiveness and sensitivity to change when considering PROMs for use in the ways envisioned for NQF-endorsed measures.

History of Successful Use of PROMs

In selecting a PROM for these various purposes, a logical first step involves reviewing what measures have already been used successfully. Using PROMs for these programs remains an understudied area, but several examples of PROMs used as indexes of performance measurement provide an initial foundation upon which the field can expand.

The Veterans Health Study assessed PROs within the Veterans Health Administration (VA) system.[326] In response to the VA's incorporation of patient-reported functional status as a domain of interest in their performance measurement system, the Veterans RAND 36-Item Health Survey (VR-36) and the Veterans Rand 12-Item Health Survey (VR-12) have been administered within the VA system to evaluate veterans' needs and to assess outcomes of clinical care at the hospital, regional, and health care system levels.[326,327] The Centers for Medicare & Medicaid Services (CMS) and its Medicare Advantage Program[328] have applied these methods for similar purposes, and CMS has also designated the VR-12 as the principal outcome measure of the Medicare Health Outcomes Survey (HOS).[329]

Research examining the VR-36 and SF-36 in such uses does inform the selection of PROs for performance measurement. Nevertheless, limitations remain to use of these measures as indicators of high-quality care and as sources of information for holding practices, providers, hospitals, health plans, or others accountable for their results. These limitations include the "static" nature of these measures, meaning that for analysts to be able to obtain an individual's score, all items must be administered—even those items that add little to the precision of measurement. In addition, content is fixed by the composition of the scale. Therefore, attention has turned to alternative PRO tools and "dynamic" instruments with clear potential for these types of uses (i.e., as patient-reported performance measures).

PROMIS constitutes arguably the best example of a future direction of PROs that will be acceptable for use in practice, quality improvement, or performance measurement programs. Developed using IRT methodology, PROMIS offers a new generation of PROMs with better reliability, validity, precision, and other attributes than is typically true for so-called legacy instruments. These measures have the important attribute of being shorter than such older instruments as well.[187] PROMIS measures form a hybrid between static generic PROMs and more flexible adaptive measures. They comprise items that are specific to the overall content of the measure but that are also applicable across the diverse spectrum of health status.

Although a growing body of literature provides preliminary evidence supporting the psychometric quality of the PROMIS measures, future work needs to explore applying PROMIS measures as tools for assessing the performance of health care organizations. Nevertheless, the PROMIS system provides a robust model by which the use of PROMs as performance measures can be expanded and elaborated upon, owing to its rigorous methodological characteristics.

Documentation of Particular Attributes of PROMs

Documentation, in peer-reviewed literature or on publicly accessible websites (or both), of the evidence of a PROM to reflect all of these measurement properties will improve acceptance of the PROM for use as a performance measure. To the extent that the evidence came from populations similar to the studies' target populations, the more confidence clinicians, analysts, administrators, and policy makers can have in the PROM to capture patients' experiences and perspectives.

Applying any set of selection standards for PROs calls for attention to several considerations. One key issue is that the populations involved in these efforts will likely be quite heterogeneous. This population heterogeneity should be reflected in the people selected to participate in the various pilot tests or studies that are part of the evaluation of the measurement properties for the PROM. For example, both qualitative and quantitative studies may require quota sampling based on race and ethnicity that reflects the prevalence of the condition in the study target population. Additionally, patients must be actively engaged as stakeholders in identifying the domains most important to measure and in selecting specific PROMs for use in performance measurement.

Participants' literacy is another important consideration for use of PROMs. Data collected from PROMs are valid only if the participants in a study can understand what is asked of them and can provide a response that accurately reflects their experiences or perspectives. Developers of PROMs must ensure that the questions and response options are clear and easy to understand. Pretesting of the instrument (e.g., cognitive testing) should include individuals with low literacy to evaluate the questions.[330]

Response burden must be considered when selecting a PROM. The instrument must not be overly burdensome for patients, as they are often sick and cannot be expected to tolerate completing lengthy questionnaires.

Finally, researchers must carefully consider the strength of evidence for the measurement properties. No threshold exists to indicate that an instrument is (or is not) valid for any or all populations or applications. In addition, no single study can confirm all the measurement properties for all contexts. Like any scientific discipline, measurement science relies on an iterative, accumulating body of evidence examining key properties in different contexts. Thus, it is the weight of the evidence that informs the evaluation of the appropriateness of a PROM. More established PROMs will have the benefit of having accrued more evidence than more recent entries; however, more recent entries tend to have improved measurement properties that warrant attention.

PROM Characteristics for Consideration

Generic Versus Condition-Specific Measures

One factor to consider when selecting a patient-level PROM is whether to use a generic instrument or a condition-specific instrument. Several considerations can inform this choice.[331] First, the specific population of interest may guide whether one opts to use a generic or condition-specific PRO. For example, if the target population comprises mainly healthy individuals, or people with multiple comorbidities, a generic measure is the preferred choice. Conversely, if the goal is to examine a specific subset of patients with a particular diagnosis or receiving a common treatment, then a condition-specific measure may be more appropriate, but this is ideally evaluated in context.

In addition, outcomes of interest may guide the selection process. Generic measures may capture a different category of outcomes when compared with a condition-specific PROM. For example, a generic measure may assess domains of general function, well-being, or quality of life, whereas a condition-specific PRO may measure symptoms expected to be directly addressed by a condition-specific intervention. The more focused the interest in a specific symptom or set of symptoms that are unique to the condition, the more likely a condition-specific instrument will be preferred.[332]

Generic PROMs have some important advantages. They allow for comparability across patients and populations,[331] although they are more suitable for comparison across groups than for individual use.[333] Global PROMs also allow assessments in terms of normative data that can be used to interpret scores.[331] This enables evaluation against population norms or comparison with information about various disease conditions. They can also be applied to individuals without specific health conditions, and they can differentiate groups on indexes of overall health and well-being.[331]

Generic PROMs also have some disadvantages. They may tend to be less responsive than condition-specific measures to focal changes that are better detected with a condition-specific measure. For that reason, they may underestimate health changes in specific patient populations.[334] Additionally, they may fail to capture important condition-specific concerns.[334]

Condition-specific PROMs are an alternative to generic PROMs. One advantage of condition-specific PROMs is the possibility for improved relevance and responsiveness.[331] They also enable differentiation of groups at the level of specific symptoms or patient concerns.[331] However, the condition-specific focus introduces the notable difficulty of making comparisons across patient populations with different diseases or health conditions.[331]

Given their respective benefits and limitations, we recommend that a combination of generic and condition-specific measures is likely to be the best choice for the performance measurement purposes that those assessing or reporting on quality of care in this country, such as the NQF, have most in mind. Generic and condition-specific PROMs may measure different aspects of HRQL when administered in combination,[335] resulting in more comprehensive assessment. Consequently, hybrid measurement systems have emerged to facilitate combining them. For example, the FACIT system consists of a generic HRQL measure plus condition-specific subscales. PROMIS, which was developed to create item banks that are appropriate for use across common chronic disease conditions,[336] represents another example of a hybrid system of PROMs that combines both global and targeted approaches.

Measurement Precision

Another factor to consider when selecting a patient-level PROM is measurement precision. Measurement precision refers to the level of variation in multiple measurements of the same factor; measures with greater precision vary less across assessment time points. PROMs with greater measurement precision also demonstrate greater sensitivity to change.[337] Given that most PROMs were originally developed as research tools, they may lack the level of precision necessary for assessing individuals on these types of outcomes.[338] Although performance measures will aggregate to practice, provider, or organization levels, adequate measurement precision at the patient level is still needed.

Regarding measurement precision, measures based on IRT tend to have greater precision than measures based on classical test theory.[338] Specifically, computerized adaptive tests (CATs) offer greater precision than static short-forms derived from item banks; however, short forms are an acceptable alternative when CAT approaches are infeasible.[339,340] Although CATs include a greater number of items in an item bank, they allow tailored measurement, resulting in shorter instruments and better precision. Consequently, using PROMs derived from IRT techniques is recommended to achieve the greatest measurement precision.

Sensitivity to Change, or Responsiveness

Sensitivity to change (also referred to as responsiveness) is another important factor to consider when selecting a PROM because the ability to detect a small, but important, change is necessary when monitoring patients and implementing clinical interventions.[38] Sensitivity to change is a type of validity characterized by within-subject changes over time following an intervention.[341,342]

Responsiveness is conceptualized in many ways, which leads to different findings and interpretations.[343] Definitions of sensitivity to change range from the ability to detect any kind of change, regardless of meaningfulness (e.g., a statistically significant change post-treatment), to the ability to detect a clinically important change. To be clinically useful, PROMs must demonstrate sensitivity to change both when individuals improve and when they deteriorate.[342]

Methods for assessing responsiveness vary markedly as well. These methods differ primarily in terms of whether they are intended to demonstrate statistically significant changes to quantify the magnitude of change.[343] The lack of equivalence across methods for detecting change can be problematic for interpretation, given that the different methods for detecting responsiveness produce different classifications of who is improved or not.[344] Indeed, relying solely on statistical tests of responsiveness is not recommended, given that such findings may not accurately reflect what is meaningful to patients or clinicians.[345]

Several factors can limit responsiveness to change. First, multi-trait scales containing items that are not relevant to the population being assessed may fail to capture change over time.[346] The responsiveness of a PROM may also be constrained by using scales that offer categorical or a limited range of response options.[346] PROMs that specify an extensive timeframe for reporting also will not be likely to demonstrate change, particularly when administered regularly over a brief period of time.[346] The responsiveness of a PROM is also limited when it includes items that reflect stable characteristics that are unlikely to change. Scales that contain items with floor or ceiling effects are also problematic.[346] A PROM sensitivity to change may depend upon the direction of the change. For example, Eurich and colleagues found that PROMs were more responsive to change when patients got better clinically than when they got worse.[38]

In addition to these factors, a growing body of research suggests that condition-specific PROMs can be more sensitive to change than generic PROMs.[38,40,347–349] Responsiveness to change is likely influenced by the purpose for which the measure was originally developed.[349] For example, measures developed to emphasize specific content areas would be expected to show greater post-treatment change in those content areas.[342] The greater sensitivity to change in condition-specific PROMs may be attributed to the strong content validity inherent in condition-specific measures.[38] As a result, using a combination of condition-specific and generic PROM may yield the most meaningful data.[38,40]

Minimally Important Differences

The difference between clinical versus statistical significance also merits consideration when selecting a PROM. Historically, research has relied upon tests of statistical significance to examine differences in scores between patients or within patients over time. However, concerns arise regarding whether statistically significant differences truly reflect differences that would be perceived as important to the patient or the clinician. Consequently, attention has shifted to the concept of clinically significant differences in PROM scores.

Experts have proposed a variety of approaches to determining clinical significance. For example, clinically significant change has been defined as "changes in patient functioning that are meaningful for individuals who undergo psychosocial or medical interventions."[350] Similarly, meaningful change is defined (from the patient perspective) as "one that results in a meaningful reduction in symptoms or improvement in function . . . ."[351]

Minimally important differences (MIDs) represent a specific approach to clinical significance. They are defined as "the smallest difference in score in the outcome of interest that informed patients or informed proxies perceive as important."[352] Minimum clinically important differences (MCIDs) constitute an even more specific category of MID. MCIDs are defined as "the smallest difference in score in the domain of interest which patients perceive as beneficial and which would mandate, in the absence of troublesome side effects and excessive cost, a change in the patient's management."[353]

Examining clinically significant differences poses several important implications.[352] First, investigating clinically significant (versus statistically significant) differences in scores aids users in interpreting PROMs. Second, focusing on clinically significant differences also emphasizes the importance of the patient perspective, which may not be adequately captured when looking mainly at statistically significant differences. Third, the ability to look at clinically significant differences in scores informs the evaluation of the success of a clinical intervention. Finally, in the context of clinical research, clinically significant differences can assist with sample size estimation.

Currently, no methodological gold standard exists for estimating MIDs.[351,354] Two primary methods are currently in use: the anchor-based method and the distribution-based method.

The anchor-based method of establishing MIDs assesses the relationship between scores on the PROM and some independent measure that is interpretable.[352] Evaluators have several options for the type of anchor they might select when using an anchor-based method. For instance, clinical anchors that are correlated with the PROM at the $r \geq 0.30$ level may serve as appropriate anchors.[304,317] Clinical trial experience can inform the selection of these clinical anchors,[355] including the use of multiple clinical anchors.[356]

Transition ratings represent another potential source of anchors when establishing MIDs. Transition ratings are patients' within-person ratings of change.[317,357] However, because of concerns about validity, experts recommend that researchers or other users examine the correlation between pre- and post-test scores and the transition rating.[358] Patients' between-person differences can also be used as anchors when establishing MIDs for PROMs.[314,317] Additional sources for anchors when establishing MIDs include HRQL-related functional measures used by clinicians[317,357] and objective standards (e.g., hospital admissions, time away from work).[358]

Although the anchor-based method offers promise for establishing MIDs in PROMs, several limitations should be considered. First, the transition rating approach to anchor selection is subject to recall bias on the part of the patient.[351] Second, global ratings may account for only some variance in scores.[351] Third, the anchor-based method does not take into consideration the measurement precision of the instruments being used.[351]

The distribution-based method represents the second method of establishing MIDs in PROMs. The distribution-based method uses the statistical characteristics of the scores when establishing MIDs.[352] Specifically, the distribution-based approach evaluates change in scores in relation to the probability that the change occurred at random.[351]

As in the case of the anchor-based method, several methods are available when applying a distribution-based approach to establishing MIDs. First, the t-test statistic has been used to establish MIDs when examining change over time.[351] However, given that this relies solely on statistical significance, it may not reflect change that is clinically meaningful, and it is also subject to variation due to sample size.[351] Second, distribution-based methods may also be grounded in measurement precision and the standard error of the mean (SEM).[351] Specifically, the 1 SEM criterion can be used as an alternative to MID when assessing the magnitude of PROM score changes.[359] Sample variation, such as effect size and standardized response mean, constitutes another method for establishing MIDs using the distribution-based method.[351] When using this method, it is recommended that the effect size be specific to the population being studied.[357] Evidence suggests that MID estimates using sample variation are approximately one-half of a standard deviation.[360]

Finally, reliable change constitutes another method of using the distribution-based approach to establish MIDs.[351] Reliable change is based on the standard error of measurement difference (SEMD); it indicates how much the observed change in an imprecise measure exceeds fluctuations that are random in nature.[351] Although the distribution-based approach serves as a possible alternative to the anchor-based methods, little consensus exists on the benchmarks for establishing changes that are clinically significant.[351]

Given limitations of the anchor- and distribution-based approaches, experts recommend that users apply multiple methods and triangulation to determine the MID.[304,351,360] Moreover, the final selection of MID values should be based on systematic review and an evaluation process such as the Delphi method.[304] MID values should also be informed by a stakeholder consensus, which includes patient engagement and input, about the extent of change considered to be meaningful. For example, in some cases, the desired outcome may be scores over time, such as in the case of interventions designed to preserve and prevent declines in functioning. Consequently, the specific application of the PRO will inform the MID values, particularly when considering the contrasts between interventions for acute clinical conditions and interventions or support for long-term or chronic conditions.

When considering MIDs for PROMs, evaluators should not apply a single MID to all situations. MIDs may vary by population and by context.[304] Consequently, those reporting such data should provide a range around the MID, rather than just a single MID value.[356] Finally, because the criteria for assessing clinically important change in individuals do not directly translate to evaluating clinically important group differences,[317] a useful strategy is to calculate the proportion of patients who experience a clinically significant change.[280,317]

Essential Conditions to Integrate PROMs Into the Electronic Health Record

General Considerations for Health Information Technology

Health information technology (HIT) has the potential to enable dramatic transformation in health care delivery. To date, however, the empirical research evidence base supporting its benefits is limited.[361]

E-health refers to health-related Internet applications that deliver a range of content, connectivity, and clinical care.[11] This includes health information, online formularies, prescription refills, appointment scheduling, test results, advance care planning and health care proxy designation, and physician-patient communication.[362] *Patient-centered e-health* (PCEH) is an emerging discipline that is defined as the combination of three themes:[363]

- Patient focus: PCEH applications are developed primarily based on needs and perspectives of patients.

- Patient activity: PCEH application designs assume that patients can participate meaningfully in providing and consuming information about, and of interest to, them.

- Patient empowerment: PCEH applications assume that patients want to, and are able to, control far-ranging aspects of their health care via a PCEH application.

Although e-health applications have become common, they tend to focus on the needs of health care providers and organizations. Patients desire a range of services to be brought online by their own health care providers.[364] However, little evidence is available as to whether the services offered by providers are services that patients desire.[12] One important consideration is that providers attend to patient acceptability factors.[12,365]

Measuring PROMs will constitute an important aspect of future stages of "meaningful use" of electronic health records (EHRs).[366,367] Access can be enhanced by allowing entry directly from commonly used devices such as smartphones. Enabling clinical decision support by providing structured data directly into EHRs will permit PROMs to be used for (1) tracking patient progress over time or (2) through individual question responses, driving change in care plans or care processes concurrently, thus improving outcomes over time. The use of a standardized instrument registered in an established code system (e.g., LOINC [Logical Observation Identifier Names and Codes]) enables EHRs to incorporate the instrument as an observation with a known set of responses using standard terminology (SNOMED-CT [Systematized Nomenclature of Medicine—Clinical Terms]) or numerical responses. Each question in the standardized instrument can also be coded (structured) to drive changes based on those responses. Unfortunately, in an updated systematic review of HIT studies published between 2004 and 2007, PROMs were not mentioned at all.[362]

The passage of the Health Information Technology for Economic and Clinical Health (HITECH) Act creates a mix of incentives and penalties that will induce a large proportion of physicians and hospitals to move toward

EHR systems by the end of the 2010s.[368] The discussion should now focus on whether HIT will support the models of care delivery that will help achieve broader policy goals: safer, more effective, and more efficient care.

Three features of EHRs are critical to enable accountable care organizations to succeed: interoperability and widespread health information exchange; automated, real-time quality and cost measurement; and smarter analytic capacities. Having a complete picture of the patient's care is a critical start, yet most EHRs are not interoperable and have limited data-sharing capabilities.[369] In summary, important issues include (1) the patient perspective (patients want to be involved "as a participant and partner in the flow of information" relating to their own health care);[370] (2) clinical buy-in; (3) compatibility with clinical flow; and (4) meaningful use.

Examples of PROMs in Electronic Health Record Applications

Health care centers are beginning to implement ways to use patient-reported information (the voice of the patient) to provide higher quality care.[371] Three recent case studies (two in the United States and one in Sweden) are particularly informative, because they illustrate lessons learned about such initiatives.[371]

The Dartmouth Spine Center collects health survey data from patients before each visit, either at home or in the clinic. Analysts summarize the data in a report and make it available for use by patients and clinicians to develop or modify care plans and to monitor results over time to guide treatment decisions. Longitudinal changes are incorporated into the report with each new assessment. At Group Health Cooperative in the State of Washington, an electronic health risk assessment has been integrated with the EHR. Patients can complete PROMs, make appointments, fill prescriptions, review health benefits, communicate with their providers, and get vetted health information. Customized reports are available to patients and providers. The Karolinska University Hospital in Stockholm, Sweden, developed a Swedish Rheumatology Quality registry in 1995 to improve the quality and value of care for people suffering from arthritis and other rheumatic diseases. Beginning in 2003, its web-based system replaced paper forms. The system uses real-time data provided by patients, clinicians, and diagnostic tests. Longitudinal summaries of PROMs and other health information are incorporated into graphical reports that are available to patients and providers.

Both patients and clinicians have generally favorable reactions to the patient-reported measurement systems implemented in these three very different health care settings. The information gathered helps to support patient-centered care by focusing attention on the health issues and outcomes that are important to patients. Although both patients and clinicians acknowledge that using PROMs takes extra time for data collection, both groups report that it makes the care more effective and efficient. Key design principles to successful use of patient-reported measurement systems include fitting PROMs into the flow of care, designing the systems with stakeholder engagement, merging data with other types of data (clinician reports, medical records, claims), and engaging in continuous improvement of the systems based on users' experiences and new technology.

Other examples include use of PROMs in managing advanced cancer where the primary goals of care are to maximize symptom management and minimize treatment toxicity. Clinicians and patients often base treatment decisions on informal assessments of HRQL. Integrating formal HRQL assessment into treatment decision making can improve patient-centered care for cancer patients with advanced disease. Computer-based assessment can reduce patient and administrative burden while enabling real-time scoring and presentation of HRQL data. Two pilot studies conducted with patients with advanced lung cancer reported that the computer technology was acceptable and feasible for patients and physicians.[167,372] Patients felt that the HRQL questionnaire helped them focus on issues to discuss with their physicians, and physicians indicated that the HRQL report helped them to evaluate patient responses over time.

A new initiative in the Robert H. Lurie Comprehensive Cancer Center at Northwestern University involves developing and implementing patient-reported symptom assessment in gynecologic oncology clinics. Before their clinic visits, outpatients complete instruments measuring fatigue, pain, physical function, depression, and anxiety through the EHR patient communication portal at home or in the clinic using an iPad. Results immediately populate the EHR. Severe symptoms trigger EHR notifications to providers. The EHR also provides automated triage for psychosocial and nutritional care when indicated.

Selection of PROMs That Meet Recommended Characteristics for Use in Performance Measures

Throughout this monograph, we have recommended several criteria that researchers and evaluators can use when assessing the appropriateness of a PROM for measuring quality of care and performance; Table 4 summarized critical points. Given that PROMs are not yet in widespread use in clinical practice, little is known about how best to aggregate these patient-level outcomes for measuring the quality of care or performance of the health care entity. Despite this limitation, accommodating the needs of patients with diverse linguistic, cultural, educational, and functional skills calls for evidence about the equivalence of multiple methods and modes of questionnaire administration. Additionally, scoring, analyzing, and reporting PRO response data all need to be user-friendly and understandable to clinicians for real-time use in clinical settings. Moreover, the timing of measurement must include administration before therapeutic interventions to allow for measuring responsiveness to change, doing risk adjustment, and screening patients for clinical intervention

To illustrate the application of these recommended characteristics when evaluating the appropriateness of a PROM for these purposes, Table 4 included one illustration of these points related to determining the success of total hip arthroplasty. Total hip arthroplasty has emerged as an acceptable surgical treatment for individuals experiencing intractable pain and severe functional impairments for whom conservative treatment has yielded minimal improvement.[373-376] The most common indication for total hip arthroplasty is joint deterioration secondary to osteoarthritis.[377] Consequently, the aging of the population is likely to raise demand for both primary total hip arthroplasty and revision procedures.[378-380]

PROs have increasingly been included alongside more traditional indices of surgical outcome such as morbidity and mortality when evaluating the success of total hip arthroplasty. With the expanding focus on patient-reported outcomes, such as functioning and quality of life, numerous, diverse PROMs have been developed and applied in measuring total hip arthroplasty outcomes.[377] Thus, this intervention provides a relevant context in which to review the use of recommended characteristics in the selection of PROMs, specifically with the characteristics of the WOMAC, a PROM developed to examine pain, stiffness, and physical function in individuals with osteoarthritis.[307]

Conclusions

PRO measures have reached a level of sophistication that enables wider use in assessing performance in clinical settings. Attention to the many methodological considerations discussed in this monograph will help users to produce meaningful, actionable results. Judicious use of a mixture of generic and condition-specific assessment instruments, acceptance of modern measurement methods such as IRT, and application of technology to enable standardized, equitable assessment across a range of patients are essential in this process. Implementing contemporary options, such as those offered by the PROMIS instruments, can effectively shorten assessment time without compromising accuracy. These attributes facilitate meeting the demands of clinical application of PROs for performance measurement.

References

1. National Quality Forum. National voluntary consensus standards for patient outcome: a consensus report. Washington, DC: NQF; 2009.

2. Lohr K, Zebrack B. Using patient-reported outcomes in clinical practice: challenges and opportunities. Qual Life Res. 2009;18(1):99-107.

3. Donaldson MS. Taking PROs and patient-centered care seriously: incremental and disruptive ideas for incorporating PROs in oncology practice. Qual Life Res. 2008;17(10):1323-30.

4. Feldman-Stewart D, Brundage MD. A conceptual framework for patient–provider communication: a tool in the PRO research tool box. Qual Life Res. 2009;18(1):109-14.

5. Greenhalgh J. The applications of PROs in clinical practice: what are they, do they work, and why? Qual Life Res. 2009;18(1):115-23.

6. Rose M, Bezjak A. Logistics of collecting patient-reported outcomes (PROs) in clinical practice: an overview and practical examples. Qual Life Res. 2009;18(1):125-36.

7. Aaronson NK, Snyder C. Using patient-reported outcomes in clinical practice: proceedings of an International Society of Quality of Life Research conference. Qual Life Res. 2008;17(10):1295-.

8. Cromwell J, Healy D, Seeley E, Trebino D, Cromwell G. The nation's health care bill: who bears the burden? Publicaton No. BK-0010-1307. Research Triangle Park, NC: RTI Press; 2013. http://dx.doi.org/10.3768/rtipress.2013.bk.0010.1307.

9. Deutsch A, Smith L, Gage B, Kelleher C, Garfinkel D. Patient-reported outcomes in performance measurement: commissioned paper on PRO-based performance measures for healthcare accountable entities. Washington, DC: National Quality Forum; 2012.

10. US Food and Drug Administration. Guidance for industry. Patient-reported outcome measures: use in medical product development to support labeling claims. 2009 [cited 2011 November 26]. Available from: http://www.fda.gov/downloads/Drugs/GuidanceComplianceRegulatory Information/Guidances/UCM071975.pdf

11. Maheu MM, Whitten P, Allen A. E-Health, telehealth, and telemedicine: a guide to start-up and success. San Francisco: Jossey-Bass; 2001.

12. Wilson EV, Lankton NK. Modeling patients' acceptance of provider-delivered e-health. J Am Med Inform Assoc. 2004;11(4):241-8.

13. Fayers P, Machin D. Quality of life: the assessment, analysis and interpretation of patient-reported outcomes. 2nd ed. Chichester: John Wiley & Sons; 2007.

14. Stephens RJ, Hopwood P, Girling DJ, Machin D. Randomized trials with quality of life endpoints: Are doctors' ratings of patients' physical symptoms interchangeable with patients' self- ratings? Qual Life Res. 1997;6(3):225-36.

15. Justice AC, Rabeneck L, Hays RD, Wu AW, Bozzette SA, for the Outcomes Committee of the ACTG. Sensitivity, specificity, reliability, and clinical validity of provider-reported symptoms: a comparison with self-reported symptoms. J Acquir Immune Defic Syndr. 1999;21(2):126-33.

16. Basch E, Iasonos A, McDonough T, Barz A, Culkin A, Kris MG, et al. Patient versus clinician symptom reporting using the National Cancer Institute Common Terminology Criteria for Adverse Events: results of a questionnaire-based study. Lancet Oncol. 2006;7(11):903-9.

17. Basch E, Jia X, Heller G, Barz A, Sit L, Fruscione M, et al. Adverse symptom event reporting by patients vs clinicians: relationships with clinical outcomes. J Natl Cancer Inst. 2009;101(23):1624-32.

18. Basch E. The missing voice of patients in drug-safety reporting. N Engl J Med. 2010;362(10):865-9.

19. Bech P. Quality of life measurements in chronic disorders. Psychother Psychosom. 1993;59(1):1-10.

20. Cella DF, Tulsky DS, Gray G, Sarafian B, Linn E, Bonomi A, et al. The Functional Assessment of Cancer Therapy scale: development and validation of the general measure. J Clin Oncol. 1993;11(3):570-9.

21. Guyatt GH. A taxonomy of health status instruments. J Rheumatol. 1995;22(6):1188-90.

22. Rothrock NE, Kaiser KA, Cella D. Developing a valid patient-reported outcome measure. Clin Pharmacol Ther. 2011;90(5):737-42.

23. Osoba D. A taxonomy of the uses of health-related quality-of-life instruments in cancer care and the clinical meaningfulness of the results. Med Care. 2002;40(6 Suppl):III31-8.

24. Benson T, Sizmur S, Whatling J, Arikan S, McDonald D, Ingram D. Evaluation of a new short generic measure of health status: howRu. Inform Prim Care. 2010;18(2):89-101.

25. Barry MJ, Fowler FJ, Jr., O'Leary MP, Bruskewitz RC, Holtgrewe HL, Mebust WK. Measuring disease-specific health status in men with benign prostatic hyperplasia. Measurement Committee of the American Urological Association. Med Care. 1995;33(4 Suppl):AS145-55.

26. Ware JE, Jr., Sherbourne CD. The MOS 36-item Short-Form Health Survey (SF-36). I. Conceptual framework and item selection. Med Care. 1992;30(6):473-83.

27. Bergner M, Bobbitt RA, Carter WB, Gilson BS. The Sickness Impact Profile: development and final revision of a health status measure. Med Care. 1981;19(8):787-805.

28. Caplan D, Hildebrandt N. Disorders of syntactic comprehension. Cambridge, Mass.: MIT Press; 1988.

29. Andresen EM, Rothenberg BM, Panzer R, Katz P, McDermott MP. Selecting a generic measure of health-related quality of life for use among older adults. A comparison of candidate instruments. Eval Health Prof. 1998;21(2):244-64.

30. Bombardier C, Melfi CA, Paul J, Green R, Hawker G, Wright J, et al. Comparison of a generic and a disease-specific measure of pain and physical function after knee replacement surgery. Med Care. 1995;33(4 Suppl):AS131-44.

31. Lundgren-Nilsson A, Tennant A, Grimby G, Sunnerhagen KS. Cross-diagnostic validity in a generic instrument: an example from the Functional Independence Measure in Scandinavia. Health Qual Life Outcomes. 2006;4:55.

32. Cella D, Yount S, Rothrock N, Gershon R, Cook K, Reeve B, et al. The Patient-Reported Outcomes Measurement Information System (PROMIS): progress of an NIH roadmap cooperative group during its first two years. Med Care. 2007;45(5 Suppl 1):S3-S11.

33. Cella D, Riley W, Stone A, Rothrock N, Reeve B, Yount S, et al. The Patient-Reported Outcomes Measurement Information System (PROMIS) developed and tested its first wave of adult self-reported health outcome item banks: 2005–2008. J Clin Epidemiol. 2010;63(11):1179-94.

34. Cella D, Lai JS, Nowinski C, Victorson D, Peterman A, Miller D, et al. Neuro-QOL: brief measures of health-related quality of life for clinical research in neurology. Neurology. 2012;78:1860-7.

35. Tulsky DS, Kisala PA, Victorson D, Tate D, Heinemann AW, Amtmann D, et al. Developing a contemporary patient-reported outcomes measure for spinal cord injury. Arch Phys Med Rehabil. 2011;92(10 Suppl):S44-S51.

36. Cella D. Manual of the Functional Assessment of Chronic Illness Therapy (FACIT Scales). Version 4 Elmhurst, IL: FACIT.org; 1997.

37. Guyatt GH, Bombardier C, Tugwell PX. Measuring disease-specific quality of life in clinical trials. Can Med Assoc J. 1986;134(8):889-95.

38. Eurich DT, Johnson JA, Reid KJ, Spertus JA. Assessing responsiveness of generic and specific health related quality of life measures in heart failure. Health Qual Life Outcomes. 2006;4:89.

39. Huang IC, Hwang CC, Wu MY, Lin W, Leite W, Wu AW. Diabetes-specific or generic measures for health-related quality of life? Evidence from psychometric validation of the D-39 and SF-36. Value Health. 2008;11(3):450-61.

40. Krahn M, Bremner KE, Tomlinson G, Ritvo P, Irvine J, Naglie G. Responsiveness of disease-specific and generic utility instruments in prostate cancer patients. Qual Life Res. 2007;16(3):509-22.

41. Cohen ME, Marino RJ. The tools of disability outcomes research functional status measures. Arch Phys Med Rehabil. 2000;81(12 Suppl 2):S21-9.

42. Bombardier C, Tugwell P. Methodological considerations in functional assessment. J Rheumatol. 1987;14(Suppl 15):6-10.

43. Gabel CP, Michener LA, Burkett B, Neller A. The Upper Limb Functional Index: development and determination of reliability, validity, and responsiveness. J Hand Ther. 2006;19(3):328-48; quiz 49.

44. Hobart J, Kalkers N, Barkhof F, Uitdehaag B, Polman C, Thompson A. Outcome measures for multiple sclerosis clinical trials: relative measurement precision of the Expanded Disability Status Scale and Multiple Sclerosis Functional Composite. Mult Scler. 2004;10(1):41-6.

45. Kaasa T, Loomis J, Gillis K, Bruera E, Hanson J. The Edmonton Functional Assessment Tool: preliminary development and evaluation for use in palliative care. J Pain Symptom Manage. 1997;13(1):10-9.

46. Mausbach BT, Moore R, Bowie C, Cardenas V, Patterson TL. A review of instruments for measuring functional recovery in those diagnosed with psychosis. Schizophr Bull. 2009;35(2):307-18.

47. Olarsch S. Validity and responsiveness of the late-life function and disability instrument in a facility-dwelling population. Boston, MA: Boston University; 2008.

48. Litwin MS, Hays R, Fink A, Ganz PA, Leake B, Brook RH. The UCLA Prostate Cancer Index: development, reliability, and validity of health-related quality of life measure. Med Care. 1998;26(7):1002-12.

49. Rosen R, Brown C, Heiman J, Leiblum S, Meston C, Shabsigh R, et al. The Female Sexual Function Index (FSFI): a multidimensional self-report instrument for the assessment of female sexual function. J Sex Marital Ther. 2000;26(2):191-208.

50. Cleeland CS. Symptom burden: multiple symptoms and their impact as patient-reported outcomes. J Natl Cancer Inst Monogr. 2007(37):16-21.

51. Smith E, Lai JS, Cella D. Building a measure of fatigue: the functional assessment of chronic illness therapy fatigue scale. PM R. 2010;2(5):359-63.

52. Yount SE, Choi SW, Victorson D, Ruo B, Cella D, Anton S, et al. Brief, valid measures of dyspnea and related functional limitations in chronic obstructive pulmonary disease (COPD). Value Health. 2011;14(2):307-15.

53. Amtmann D, Cook KF, Jensen MP, Chen W-H, Choi S, Revicki D, et al. Development of a PROMIS item bank to measure pain interference. Pain. 2010;150(1):173-82.

54. Centers for Disease Control and Prevention (CDC). Workplace health promotion-glossary terms 2012 [cited 2012 September 25]. Available from: http://www.cdc.gov/workplacehealthpromotion/glossary/#H.

55. Oremus M, Hammill A, Raina P. Health risk appraisal, technology assessment report. Rockville, MD: US Agency for Healthcare Research and Quality; 2011.

56. Wellsource Inc. Scientific validity 2011 [cited 2012 September 25]. Available from: www.wellsource.com/scientific-validity.html.

57. Goetzel RZ, Ozminkowski RJ, Bruno JA, Rutter KR, Isaac F, Wang S. The long-term impact of Johnson & Johnson's Health & Wellness Program on employee health risks. J Occup Environ Med. 2002;44(5):417-24.

58. Centers for Disease Control and Prevention (CDC). Behavioral Risk Factor Surveillance System 2012 [cited 2012 September 11]. Available from: http://www.cdc.gov/brfss.

59. Centers for Disease Control and Prevention (CDC). National Health and Nutrition Examination Survey, 2007-2008: overview. Hyattsville, MD: CDC National Center for Health Statistics; 2008.

60. Bonevski B, Campbell E, Sanson-Fisher RW. The validity and reliability of an interactive computer tobacco and alcohol use survey in general practice. Addict Behav. 2010;35(5):492-8.

61. Couwenbergh C, van der Gaag RJ, Koeter M, de Ruiter C, van den Brink W. Screening for substance abuse among adolescents validity of the CAGE-AID in youth mental health care. Subst Use Misuse. 2009;44(6):823-34.

62. Paxton AE, Strycker LA, Toobert DJ, Ammerman AS, Glasgow RE. Starting the conversation performance of a brief dietary assessment and intervention tool for health professionals. Am J Prev Med. 2011;40(1):67-71.

63. Sallis R. Developing healthcare systems to support exercise: exercise as the fifth vital sign. Br J Sports Med. 2011;45(6):473-4.

64. Wong SL, Leatherdale ST, Manske SR. Reliability and validity of a school-based physical activity questionnaire. Med Sci Sports Exerc. 2006;38(9):1593-600.

65. Morisky DE, Ang A, Krousel-Wood M, Ward HJ. Predictive validity of a medication adherence measure in an outpatient setting. J Clin Hypertens. 2008;10(5):348-54.

66. Agency for Healthcare Research and Quality (US). Notice number: NOT-HS-05-005. Special emphasis notice: research priorities for the Agency for Healthcare Research and Quality 2005 [cited 2012 June 25]. Available from: http://grants.nih.gov/grants/guide/notice-files/NOT-HS-05-005.html.

67. Institute of Medicine. Crossing the quality chasm: a new health system for the 21st century. Washington, DC: National Academy Press; 2001.

68. Hall JA, Dornan MC. Meta-analysis of satisfaction with medical care: Description of research domain and analysis of overall satisfaction levels. Soc Sci Med. 1988;27(6):637-44.

69. Lewis JR. Patient views on quality care in general practice: literature review. Soc Sci Med. 1994;39(5):655-70.

70. Locker D, Dunt D. Theoretical and methodological issues in sociological studies of consumer satisfaction with medical care. Soc Sci Med. 1978;12:283-92.

71. Pascoe GC. Patient satisfaction in primary health care: a literature review and analysis. Eval Program Plann. 1983;6(3-4):185-210.

72. Williams B. Patient satisfaction: a valid concept? Soc Sci Med. 1994;38(4):509-16.

73. Shikiar R, Rentz AM. Satisfaction with medication: an overview of conceptual, methodologic, and regulatory issues. Value Health. 2004;7(2):204-15.

74. Linder-Pelz SU. Toward a theory of patient satisfaction. Soc Sci Med. 1982;16(5):577-82.

75. Oberst MT. Patients' perceptions of care. Measurement of quality and satisfaction. Cancer. 1984;53(10):2366-75.

76. National Quality Forum (NQF). Safe practices for better healthcare–2010 update. Washington, DC: NQF; 2010.

77. Ware JE, Jr., Snyder MK, Wright WR, Davies AR. Defining and measuring patient satisfaction with medical care. Eval Program Plann. 1983;6(3-4):247-63.

78. Cella D, Bonomi A, Leslie WT, VonRoenn J, Tchekmedyian NS. Quality of life and nutritional well-being: measurement and relationship. Oncology. 1993;7(11, Suppl):S105-S11.

79. Rubin HR, Gandek B, Rogers WH, Kosinski M, McHorney CA, Ware JE, Jr. Patients' ratings of outpatient visits in different practice settings. Results from the Medical Outcomes Study. JAMA. 1993;270(7):835-40.

80. Graham J. Foundation for accountability(FACCT): a major new voice in the quality debate. In: Boyle J, editor. 1997 Medical Outcomes & Guidelines Sourcebook: a progress report and resource guide on medical outcomes research and practice guidelines: developments, data, and documentation. New York: Faulkner & Gray; 1996.

81. Hays RD, Davies AR, Ware JE. Scoring the Medical Outcomes Study Patient Satisfaction Questionnaire: PSQ-III. MOS memorandum No. 866. Santa Monica, CA: Rand Corp; 1987.

82. Moinpour CM. Assessment of quality of life in clinical trials. Quality of life assesment in cancer clinical trials. Report of the Workshop on Quality of Life Research in Cancer Clinical Trials, July 16-17, 1990. Bethesda, MD: US Department of Health and Human Services; 1991.

83. Williams S. Consumer satisfaction surveys: health plan report cards to guide consumers in selecting benefit programs. In: Boyle J, editor. 1997 Medical Outcomes & Guidelines Sourcebook: a progress report and resource guide on medical outcomes research and practice guidelines: developments, data, and documentation. New York: Faulkner & Gray; 1996.

84. Speight J. Assessing patient satisfaction: concepts, applications, and measurement. Value Health. 2005;8 Suppl 1:S6-8.

85. Epstein LH, Cluss PA. A behavioral medicine perspective on adherence to long-term medical regimens. J Consult Clin Psychol. 1982;50(6):950-71.

86. Sherbourne CD, Hays RD, Ordway L, DiMatteo MR, Kravitz RL. Antecedents of adherence to medical recommendations: Results from the Medical Outcomes Study. J Behav Med. 1992;15(5):447-68.

87. Hays RD, Kravitz RL, Mazel RM, Sherbourne CD, DiMatteo MR, Rogers WH, et al. The impact of patient adherence on health outcomes for patients with chronic disease in the Medical Outcomes Study. J Behav Med. 1994;17(4):347-60.

88. Hirsh AT, Atchison JW, Berger JJ, Waxenberg LB, Lafayette-Lucey A, Bulcourf BB, et al. Patient satisfaction with treatment for chronic pain: predictors and relationship to compliance. Clin J Pain. 2005;21(4):302-10.

89. Ickovics JR, Meisler AW. Adherence in AIDS clinical trials: a framework for clinical research and clinical care. J Clin Epidemiol. 1997;50(4):385-91.

90. Kincey J, Bradshaw P, Ley P. Patients' satisfaction and reported acceptance of advice in general practice. J R Coll Gen Pract. 1975;25(157):558-66.

91. Augustin M, Reich C, Schaefer I, Zschocke I, Rustenbach SJ. Development and validation of a new instrument for the assessment of patient-defined benefit in the treatment of acne. Journal der Deutschen Dermatologischen Gesellschaft. 2008;6(2):113-20.

92. Blais MA. Development of an inpatient treatment alliance scale. J Nerv Ment Dis. 2004;192(7):487-93.

93. Brod M, Christensen T, Bushnell D. Maximizing the value of validation findings to better understand treatment satisfaction issues for diabetes. Qual Life Res. 2007;16(6):1053-63.

94. Flood EM, Beusterien KM, Green H, Shikiar R, Baran RW, Amonkar MM, et al. Psychometric evaluation of the Osteoporosis Patient Treatment Satisfaction Questionnaire (OPSAT-Q), a novel measure to assess satisfaction with bisphosphonate treatment in postmenopausal women. Health Qual Life Outcomes. 2006;4:42.

95. Hudak PL, Hogg-Johnson S, Bombardier C, McKeever PD, Wright JG. Testing a new theory of patient satisfaction with treatment outcome. Med Care. 2004;42(8):726-39.

96. Kumar RN, Kirking DM, Hass SL, Vinokur AD, Taylor SD, Atkinson MJ, et al. The association of consumer expectations, experiences and satisfaction with newly prescribed medications. Qual Life Res. 2007;16(7):1127-36.

97. Pouchot J, Trudeau E, Hellot SC, Meric G, Waeckel A, Goguel J. Development and psychometric validation of a new patient satisfaction instrument: the osteoARthritis Treatment Satisfaction (ARTS) questionnaire. Qual Life Res. 2005;14(5):1387-99.

98. Taback NA, Bradley C. Validation of the genital herpes treatment satisfaction questionnaire (GHerpTSQ) in status and change versions. Qual Life Res. 2006;15(6):1043-52.

99. Cella DF. Quality of life: the concept. J Palliat Care. 1992;8(3):8-13.

100. Wagner EH. Chronic disease management: what will it take to improve care for chronic illness? Eff Clin Pract. 1998;1(1):2-4.

101. Greene J, Hibbard JH. Why does patient activation matter? An examination of the relationships between patient activation and health-related outcomes. J Gen Intern Med. 2012;27(5):520-6.

102. Hibbard JH, Greene J. What the evidence shows about patient activation: better health outcomes and care experiences; fewer data on costs. Health Aff (Millwood). 2013;32(2):207-14.

103. Hibbard JH, Stockard J, Mahoney ER, Tusler M. Development of the Patient Activation Measure (PAM): conceptualizing and measuring activation in patients and consumers. Health Serv Res. 2004;39(4p1):1005-26.

104. Hibbard JH. Using systematic measurement to target consumer activation strategies. Med Care Res Rev. 2009;66(1 suppl):9S-27S.

105. Hibbard JH, Mahoney ER, Stock R, Tusler M. Do increases in patient activation result in improved self-management behaviors? Health Serv Res. 2007;42(4):1443-63.

106. Lake T, Kvan C, Gold M. Literature review: using quality information for health care decisions and quality improvement. Mathematica Policy Research. 2005;Reference No. 6110-230.

107. Schneider EC, Zaslavsky AM, Landon BE, Lied TR, Sheingold S, Cleary PD. National quality monitoring of Medicare health plans: the relationship between enrollees' reports and the quality of clinical care. Med Care. 2001;39(12):1313-25.

108. Browne K, Roseman D, Shaller D, Edgman-Levitan S. Analysis & commentary. Measuring patient experience as a strategy for improving primary care. Health Aff (Millwood). 2010;29(5):921-5.

109. Cella DF, Lloyd SR. Data collection strategies for patient-reported information. Qual Manag Health Care. 1994;2(4):28-35.

110. Sneeuw KC, Sprangers MA, Aaronson NK. The role of health care providers and significant others in evaluating the quality of life of patients with chronic disease. J Clin Epidemiol. 2002;55(11):1130-43.

111. Eiser C, Morse R. A review of measures of quality of life for children with chronic illness. Arch Dis Child. 2001;84(3):205-11.

112. Eiser C, Morse R. Quality-of-life measures in chronic diseases of childhood. Health Technol Assess. 2001;5(4):1-157.

113. Weinfurt KP, Trucco SM, Willke RJ, Schulman KA. Measuring agreement between patient and proxy responses to multidimensional health-related quality-of-life measures in clinical trials. An application of psychometric profile analysis. J Clin Epidemiol. 2002;55(6):608-18.

114. Andresen EM, Vahle VJ, Lollar D. Proxy reliability: Health-related quality of life (HRQoL) measures for people with disability. Qual Life Res. 2001;10(7):609-19.

115. Hart T, Whyte J, Polansky M, Millis S, Hammond FM, Sherer M, et al. Concordance of patient and family report of neurobehavioral symptoms at 1 year after traumatic brain injury. Arch Phys Med Rehabil. 2003;84(2):204-13.

116. Matziou V, Perdikaris P, Feloni D, Moshovi M, Tsoumakas K, Merkouris A. Cancer in childhood: children's and parents' aspects for quality of life. Eur J Oncol Nurs. 2008;12(3):209-16.

117. Matziou V, Tsoumakas K, Perdikaris P, Feloni D, Moschovi M, Merkouris A. Corrigendum to: "Cancer in childhood: children's and parents' aspects for quality of life" [Eur J Oncol Nurs 12 (2008) 209-216] (DOI:10.1016/j. ejon.2007.10.005). Eur J Oncol Nurs. 2009;13(5).

118. Oczkowski C, O'Donnell M. Reliability of proxy respondents for patients with stroke: a systematic review. J Stroke Cerebrovasc Dis. 2010;19(5):410-6.

119. Brown-Jacobsen AM, Wallace DP, Whiteside SPH. Multimethod, multi-informant agreement, and positive predictive value in the identification of child anxiety disorders using the SCAS and ADIS-C. Assessment. 2011;18(3):382-92.

120. Agnihotri K, Awasthi S, Singh U, Chandra H, Thakur S. A study of concordance between adolescent self-report and parent-proxy report of health-related quality of life in school-going adolescents. J Psychosom Res. 2010;69(6):525-32.

121. Dorman PJ, Waddell F, Slattery J, Dennis M, Sandercock P. Are proxy assessments of health status after stroke with the EuroQol questionnaire feasible, accurate, and unbiased? Stroke. 1997;28(10):1883-7.

122. Duncan PW, Lai SM, Tyler D, Perera S, Reker DM, Studenski S. Evaluation of proxy responses to the Stroke Impact Scale. Stroke. 2002;33(11):2593-9.

123. Ostbye T, Tyas S, McDowell I, Koval J. Reported activities of daily living: agreement between elderly subjects with and without dementia and their caregivers. Age Ageing. 1997;26(2):99-106.

124. Sneeuw KC, Aaronson NK, de Haan RJ, Loeb JM. Assessing quality of life after stroke. The value and limitations of proxy ratings. Stroke. 1997;28(8):1541-9.

125. Morrow AM, Hayen A, Quine S, Scheinberg A, Craig JC. A comparison of doctors', parents' and children's reports of health states and health-related quality of life in children with chronic conditions. Child Care Health Dev. 2012;38(2):186-95.

126. White-Koning M, Arnaud C, Dickinson HO, Thyen U, Beckung E, Fauconnier J, et al. Determinants of child-parent agreement in quality-of-life reports: a European study of children with cerebral palsy. Pediatrics. 2007;120(4):804-14.

127. Upton P, Lawford J, Eiser C. Parent-child agreement across child health-related quality of life instruments: a review of the literature. Qual Life Res. 2008;17(6):895-913.

128. Hilari K, Owen S, Farrelly SJ. Proxy and self-report agreement on the Stroke and Aphasia Quality of Life Scale-39. J Neurol Neurosurg Psychiatry. 2007;78(10):1072-5.

129. Lynn Snow A, Cook KF, Lin P-S, Morgan RO, Magaziner J. Proxies and Other External Raters: Methodological Considerations. Health Serv Res. 2005;40(5p2):1676-93.

130. Fowler FJ, Jr. Data collection methods. In: Spilker B, editor. Quality of life and pharmacoeconomics in clinical trials. 2nd edition. Philadelphia: Lippincott-Raven Publishers; 1996.

131. Naughton MJ, Shumaker SA, Anderson RT, Czajkowski SM. Psychological aspects of health-related quality of life measurement: tests and scales. In: Spilker B, editor. Quality of life and pharmacoeconomics in clinical trials. 2nd edition Philadelphia: Lippincott-Raven; 1996.

132. Groves RM. Survey methodology. 2nd ed. Hoboken, NJ: J. Wiley; 2009.

133. Selltiz C, Wrightsman LS, Cook SW. Research methods in social relations. New York: Holt, Rinehart and Winston; 1976.

134. Edwards AL. Techniques of attitude scale construction. New York: Appleton-Century-Crofts; 1957.

135. Crowne DP, Marlowe D. The approval motive: studies in evaluative dependence. New York: Wiley; 1964.

136. Bowling A. Mode of questionnaire administration can have serious effects on data quality. J Public Health. 2005;27(3):281-91.

137. Anderson JP, Bush JW, Berry CC. Classifying function for health outcome and quality-of-life evaluation. Self- versus interviewer modes. Med Care. 1986;24(5):454-69.

138. Cook DJ, Guyatt GH, Juniper E, Griffith L, McIlroy W, Willan A, et al. Interviewer versus self-administered questionnaires in developing a disease-specific, health-related quality of life instrument for asthma. J Clin Epidemiol. 1993;46(6):529-34.

139. McHorney CA, Kosinski M, Ware JE, Jr. Comparisons of the costs and quality of norms for the SF-36 health survey collected by mail versus telephone interview: results from a national survey. Med Care. 1994;32(6):551-67.

140. Chan KS, Orlando M, Ghosh-Dastidar B, Duan N, Sherbourne CD. The interview mode effect on the Center for Epidemiological Studies Depression (CES-D) scale: an item response theory analysis. Med Care. 2004;42(3):281-9.

141. Weinberger M, Oddone EZ, Samsa GP, Landsman PB. Are health-related quality-of-life measures affected by the mode of administration? J Clin Epidemiol. 1996;49(2):135-40.

142. Chambers LW, Haight M, Norman G, MacDonald L. Sensitivity to change and the effect of mode of administration on health status measurement. Med Care. 1987;25(6):470-80.

143. Wu AW, Jacobson DL, Berzon RA, Revicki DA, van der Horst C, Fichtenbaum CJ, et al. The effect of mode of administration on medical outcomes study health ratings and EuroQol scores in AIDS. Qual Life Res. 1997;6(1):3-10.

144. Teresi JA. Overview of quantitative measurement methods: equivalence, invariance, and differential item functioning in health applications. Med Care. 2006;44(11 Suppl 3):S39-S49.

145. Teresi JA. Different approaches to differential item functioning in health applications: advantages, disadvantages and some neglected topics. Med Care. 2006;44(11 Suppl 3):S152-S70.

146. Borsboom D. When does measurement invariance matter? Med Care. 2006;44(11 Suppl 3):S176-S81.

147. Hambleton RK. Good practices for identifying differential item functioning. Med Care. 2006;44(11 Suppl 3):S182-S8.

148. McHorney CA, Fleishman JA. Assessing and understanding measurement equivalence in health outcome measures: issues for further quantitative and qualitative inquiry. Med Care. 2006;44(11 Suppl 3):S205-S10.

149. Coons SJ, Gwaltney CJ, Hays RD, Lundy JJ, Sloan JA, Revicki DA, et al. Recommendations on evidence needed to support measurement equivalence between electronic and paper-based patient-reported outcome (PRO) measures: ISPOR ePRO Good Research Practices Task Force report. Value Health. 2009;12(4):419-29.

150. Hahn E, Cella D, Dobrez D, Shiomoto G, Marcus E, Taylor SG, et al. The talking touchscreen: a new approach to outcomes assessment in low literacy. Psychooncology. 2004;13(2):86-95.

151. Hahn EA, Cella D, Dobrez DG, Shiomoto G, Taylor SG, Galvez AG, et al. Quality of life assessment for low literacy Latinos: a new multimedia program for self-administration. J Oncol Manag. 2003;12(5):9-12.

152. Greist JH, Klein MH, Van Cura LJ, Erdman HP. Computer interview questionnaires for drug use/abuse, p. 164-74. In: Lettieri DJ, editor. Predicting adolescent drug abuse: a review of issues, methods and correlates. Bethesda, MD: National Institute on Drug Abuse; 1975. Available from: US Government Printing Office, Washington, DC: Publication Number (ADM) 76-299.

153. Gwaltney CJ, Shields AL, Shiffman S. Equivalence of electronic and paper-and-pencil administration of patient-reported outcome measures: a meta-analytic review. Value Health. 2008;11(2):322-33.

154. Dalal AA, Nelson L, Gilligan T, McLeod L, Lewis S, DeMuro-Mercon C. Evaluating patient-reported outcome measurement comparability between paper and alternate versions, using the lung function questionnaire as an example. Value Health. 2011;14(5):712-20.

155. Abernethy AP, Herndon JE, Wheeler JL, Patwardhan M, Shaw H, Lyerly HK, et al. Improving health care efficiency and quality using tablet personal computers to collect research-quality, patient-reported data. Health Serv Res. 2008;43(6):1975-91.

156. Abernethy AP, Zafar SY, Wheeler JL, Lyerly HK, Ahmad A, Reese JB. Electronic patient-reported data capture as a foundation of rapid learning cancer care. Med Care. 2010;48(6 suppl.):S32-S8.

157. Dudgeon D, King S, Howell D, Green E, Gilbert J, Hughes E, et al. Cancer Care Ontario's experience with implementation of routine physical and psychological symptom distress screening. Psychooncology. 2012;21(4):357-64.

158. Gilbert JE, Howell D, King S, Sawka C, Hughes E, Angus H, et al. Quality improvement in cancer symptom assessment and control: the Provincial Palliative Care Integration Project (PPCIP). J Pain Symptom Manage. 2012;43(4):663-78.

159. Snyder CF, Jensen R, Courtin SO, Wu AW. PatientViewpoint: a website for patient-reported outcomes assessment. Qual Life Res. 2009;18(7):793-800.

160. Velikova G, Booth L, Smith AB, Brown PM, Lynch P, Brown JM, et al. Measuring quality of life in routine oncology practice improves communication and patient well-being: a randomized controlled trial. J Clin Oncol. 2004;22(4):714-24.

161. Detmar SB, Muller MJ, Schornagel JH, Wever LD, Aaronson NK. Health-related quality-of-life assessments and patient-physician communication: a randomized controlled trial. JAMA. 2002;288(23):3027-34.

162. Velikova G, Brown JM, Smith AB, Selby PJ. Computer-based quality of life questionnaires may contribute to doctor-patient interactions in oncology. Br J Cancer. 2002;86(1):51-9.

163. Suh SY, Leblanc TW, Shelby RA, Samsa GP, Abernethy AP. Longitudinal patient-reported performance status assessment in the cancer clinic is feasible and prognostic. J Oncol Pract. 2011;7(6):374-81.

164. Fihn SD, Bucher JB, McDonell M. Collaborative care intervention for stable ischemic heart disease. Arch Intern Med. 2011;171(16):1471-9.

165. Fihn SD, McDonell MB, Diehr P, Anderson SM, Bradley KA, Au DH, et al. Effects of sustained audit/feedback on self-reported health status of primary care patients. Am J Med. 2004;116(4):241-8.

166. Au DH, McDonell MB, Martin DC, Fihn SD. Regional variations in health status. Med Care. 2001;39(8):879-88.

167. Chang CH, Cella D, Masters GA, Laliberte N, O'Brien P, Peterman A, et al. Real-time clinical application of quality-of-life assessment in advanced lung cancer. Clin Lung Cancer. 2002;4(2):104-9.

168. Wright EP, Selby PJ, Crawford M, Gillibrand A, Johnston C, Perren TJ, et al. Feasibility and compliance of automated measurement of quality of life in oncology practice. J Clin Oncol. 2003;21(2):374-82.

169. Valderas J, Kotzeva A, Espallargues M, Guyatt G, Ferrans C, Halyard M, et al. The impact of measuring patient-reported outcomes in clinical practice: a systematic review of the literature. Qual Life Res. 2008;17(2):179-93.

170. Marshall S, Haywood K, Fitzpatrick R. Impact of patient-reported outcome measures on routine practice: a structured review. J Eval Clin Pract. 2006;12(5):559-68.

171. Mullen KH, Berry DL, Zierler BK. Computerized symptom and quality-of-life assessment for patients with cancer part II: acceptability and usability. Oncol Nurs Forum. 2004;31(5):E84-E9.

172. Jones JB, Snyder CF, Wu AW. Issues in the design of Internet-based systems for collecting patient-reported outcomes. Qual Life Res. 2007;16(8):1407-17.

173. Cleeland CS, Wang XS, Shi Q, Mendoza TR, Wright SL, Berry MD, et al. Automated symptom alerts reduce postoperative symptom severity after cancer surgery: a randomized controlled clinical trial. J Clin Oncol. 2011;29(8):994-1000.

174. Basch E, Artz D, Iasonos A, Speakman J, Shannon K, Lin K, et al. Evaluation of an online platform for cancer patient self-reporting of chemotherapy toxicities. J Am Med Inform Assoc. 2007;14(3):264-8.

175. Hardwick ME, Pulido PA, Adelson WS. The use of handheld technology in nursing research and practice. Orthop Nurs. 2007;26(4):251-5.

176. Bollen K, Lennox R. Conventional wisdom on measurement: A structural equation perspective. Psychol Bull. 1991;110(2):305-14.

177. MacCallum RC, Browne MW. The use of causal indicators in covariance structure models: some practical issues. Psychol Bull. 1993;114(3):533-41.

178. Fayers PM, Hand DJ. Factor analysis, causal indicators and quality of life. Qual Life Res. 1997;6(2):139-50.

179. Fayers PM, Hand DJ, Bjordal K, Groenvold M. Causal indicators in quality of life research. Qual Life Res. 1997;6(5):393-406.

180. Sebille V, Hardouin J-B, Le Neel T, Kubis G, Boyer F, Guillemin F, et al. Methodological issues regarding power of classical test theory (CTT) and item response theory (IRT)-based approaches for the comparison of patient-reported outcomes in two groups of patients--a simulation study. BMC Med Res Methodol. 2010;10:24.

181. Bjorner JB, Chang C-H, Thissen D, Reeve BB. Developing tailored instruments: item banking and computerized adaptive assessment. Qual Life Res. 2007;16(Suppl1):95-108.

182. Cook KF, O'Malley KJ, Roddey TS. Dynamic assessment of health outcomes: time to let the CAT out of the bag? Health Serv Res. 2005;40(5 Pt 2):1694-711.

183. Cook KF, Teal CR, Bjorner JB, Cella D, Chang CH, Crane PK, et al. IRT health outcomes data analysis project: an overview and summary. Qual Life Res. 2007;16 Suppl 1:121-32.

184. Coster W, Ludlow L, Mancini M. Using IRT variable maps to enrich understanding of rehabilitation data. J Outcome Meas. 1999;3(2):123-33.

185. Edelen MO, Reeve BB. Applying item response theory (IRT) modeling to questionnaire development, evaluation, and refinement. Qual Life Res. 2007;16 Suppl 1:5-18.

186. Fayers PM. Applying item response theory and computer adaptive testing: the challenges for health outcomes assessment. Qual Life Res. 2007;16 Suppl 1:187-94.

187. Fries JF, Bruce B, Cella D. The promise of PROMIS: using item response theory to improve assessment of patient-reported outcomes. Clin Exp Rheumatol. 2005;23(S38):S33-S7.

188. Pallant JF, Tennant A. An introduction to the Rasch measurement model: an example using the Hospital Anxiety and Depression Scale (HADS). Br J Clin Psychol. 2007;46(Pt 1):1-18.

189. Reeve BB, Hays RD, Bjorner JB, Cook KF, Crane PK, Teresi JA, et al. Psychometric evaluation and calibration of health-related quality of life item banks: plans for the Patient-Reported Outcomes Measurement Information System (PROMIS). Med Care. 2007;45(5 Suppl 1):S22-S31.

190. Nunnally JC, Bernstein IH. Psychometric Theory. New York: McGraw-Hill, Inc.; 1994.

191. Fleiss JL. The design and analysis of clinical experiments. New York: John Wiley & Sons; 1986.

192. Lord FM, Novick MR. Statistical theories of mental test scores. Reading, MA: Addison-Wesley 1968.

193. Allen MJ, Yen WM. Introduction to measurement theory. Monterey, CA: Brooks/Cole Publishing; 1979.

194. DeVellis RF. Classical test theory. Med Care. 2006;44(11 Suppl 3):S50-S9.

195. DeVellis RF. Scale development theory and applications. Thousand Oaks, CA: Sage; 2003.

196. Martinez-Martin P. Composite rating scales. J Neurol Sci. 2010;289(1-2):7-11.

197. Streiner DL, Norman GR. Health measurement scales. A practical guide to their development and use. New York: Oxford University Press; 2003.

198. Hambleton RK, Swaminathan H, Rogers HJ. Fundamentals of item response theory. Newbury Park, CA: SAGE Publications, Inc.; 1991.

199. Hambleton RK. Emergence of item response modeling in instrument development and data analysis. Med Care. 2000;38(9 Suppl):II60-II5.

200. van der Linden WJ, Hambleton RK. Handbook of modern item response theory. New York: Springer-Verlag; 1997.

201. Wright BD, Masters GN. Rating scale analysis: Rasch measurement. Chicago: MESA Press; 1985.

202. Cook KF, Monahan PO, McHorney CA. Delicate balance between theory and practice: health status assessment and item response theory. Med Care. 2003;41(5):571-4.

203. McHorney CA, Cohen AS. Equating health status measures with item response theory: Illustrations with functional status items. Med Care. 2000;38(9 Suppl):1143-59.

204. Dorans N. Comparing or combining scores from multiple instruments: instrument linking (equating). Presented at: Advances in Health Outcomes Measurement: Exploring the Current State and the Future of Item Response Theory, Item Banks, and Computer-Adaptive Testing; 2004 Jun 24-25; Bethesda, MD.

205. Quality First: Better Health Care for All Americans. Final Report of the President's Advisory Commission on Consumer Protection and Quality in the Health Care Industry. Washington, DC: US Government Printing Office, 1998.

206. Hahn EA, Cella D. Health outcomes assessment in vulnerable populations: measurement challenges and recommendations. Arch Phys Med Rehabil. 2003;84(Suppl 2):S35-S42.

207. Agency for Healthcare Research Quality. National healthcare disparities report 2010. Rockville, MD: US Agency for Healthcare Research and Quality; 2011.

208. Hahn E, Cella D, Dobrez D, Weiss B, Du H, Lai JS, et al. The impact of literacy on health-related quality of life measurement and outcomes in cancer outpatients. Qual Life Res. 2007;16(3):495-507.

209. Kirsch I, Jungeblut A, Jenkins L, Kolstad A. Adult literacy in America: a first look at the results of the National Adult Literacy Survey. Washington, DC: National Center for Education Statistics, US Department of Education; 1993.

210. Kutner M. National Center for Education Statistics. Literacy in everyday life: results from the 2003 National Assessment of Adult Literacy (NCES 2007–480). US Department of Education. Washington, DC: National Center for Education Statistics; 2007.

211. DeWalt DA, Berkman ND, Sheridan S, Lohr KN, Pignone MP. Literacy and health outcomes: a systematic review of the literature. J Gen Intern Med. 2004;19(12):1228-39.

212. Berkman ND, Sheridan SL, Donahue KE, Halpern DJ, Crotty K. Low health literacy and health outcomes: an updated systematic review. Ann Intern Med. 2011;155:97-107.

213. US Department of Health and Human Services. Healthy people 2010: understanding and improving health, 2nd ed. Washington, DC: US Government Printing Office; 2000.

214. Committee on Health Literacy, Nielsen-Bohlman L, Panzer AM, Kindig DA. Health literacy: a prescription to end confusion. Washington, DC: National Academies Press; 2004.

215. Berkman ND, Sheridan SL, Donahue KE, Halpern DJ, Viera A, Crotty K, et al. Health literacy interventions and outcomes: an updated systematic

review, executive summary. Evidence Report/Technology Assessment No. 199. Rockville, MD: US Agency for Healthcare Research and Quality, 2011 March. Report No. 11-E006-1.

216. Kutner M, Greenberg E, Jin Y, Paulsen C. The health literacy of America's adults: results from the 2003 National Assessment of Adult Literacy (NCES 2006–483). Washington, DC: National Center for Education Statistics: US Department of Education; 2006.

217. Baker DW, Gazmararian JA, Williams MV, Scott T, Parker RM, Green D, et al. Functional health literacy and the risk of hospital admission among Medicare managed care enrollees. Am J Public Health. 2002;92(8):1278-83.

218. Rudd RE, Anderson JE, Oppenheimer S, Nath C. Health literacy: an update of public health and medical literature. In: Comings JP, Garner B, Smith CA, editors. Review of adult learning and literacy. 7. Mahwah, NJ: Lawrence Erlbaum Associates; 2007. p. 175-204.

219. Macabasco-O'Connell A, DeWalt D, Broucksou K, Hawk V, Baker D, Schillinger D, et al. Relationship between literacy, knowledge, self-care behaviors, and heart failure-related quality of life among patients with heart failure. J Gen Intern Med. 2011:1-8.

220. Ad Hoc Committee on Health Literacy for the Council on Scientific Affairs, American Medical Association. Health literacy: report of the Council on Scientific Affairs. JAMA. 1999;281(6):552-7.

221. Parikh NS, Parker RM, Nurss JR, Baker DW, Williams MV. Shame and health literacy: the unspoken connection. Patient Educ Couns. 1996;27(1):33-9.

222. Baker DW, Parker RM, Williams MV, Coates WC, Pitkin K. Use and effectiveness of interpreters in an emergency department. JAMA. 1996;274(10):783-8.

223. Lennon C, Burdick H. The Lexile framework as an approach for reading measurement and success. Durham, NC: MetaMetrics; 2004. Available from: https://cdn.lexile.com/cms_page_media/135/The%20Lexile%20 Framework%20for%20Reading.pdf

224. Klare GR. The measurement of readability. Ames: Iowa State University Press; 1963.

225. Liberman IY, Mann VA, Shankweiler D, Werfelman M. Children's memory for recurring linguistic and nonlinguistic material in relation to reading ability. Cortex. 1982;18(3):367-75.

226. Shankweiler D, Crain S. Language mechanisms and reading disorder: a modular approach. Cognition. 1986;24(1-2):139-68.

227. Crain S, Shankweiler D. Syntactic Complexity and Reading Acquisition. In: Davidson A, Green GM, editors. Linguistic complexity and text comprehension: readability issues reconsidered. Hillsdale, NJ: Lawrence Erlbaum Associates, Inc; 1988. p. 167-92.

228. Brach C, Keller D, Hernandez LM, Baur C, Parker R, Dreyer B, et al. Ten attributes of health literate health care organizations. Washington, DC: National Academies Press; 2012.

229. US Department of Health and Human Services Office of Minority Health. National standards for culturally and linguistically appropriate services in health care. Washington, DC: US Department of Health and Human Services; 2001.

230. Drasgow F, Kanfer R. Equivalence of psychological measurement in heterogeneous populations. J Appl Psychol. 1985;70:662-80.

231. Hui CH, Triandis HC. Measurement in cross-cultural psychology. J Cross Cult Psychol. 1985;16(2):131-52.

232. Angel R, Thoits P. The impact of culture on the cognitive structure of illness. Cult Med Psychiatry. 1987;11 23-52.

233. Bullinger M, Anderson R, Cella D, Aaronson N. Developing and evaluating cross-cultural instruments from minimum requirements to optimal models. Qual Life Res. 1993;2(6):451-9.

234. Hayes RP, Baker DW. Methodological problems in comparing English-speaking and Spanish-speaking patients' satisfaction with interpersonal aspects of care. Med Care. 1998;36(2):230-6.

235. Bjorner JB, Thunedborg K, Kristensen TS, Modvig J, Bech P. The Danish SF-36 health survey: translation and preliminary validity studies. J Clin Epidemiol. 1998;51(11):991-9.

236. Hunt SM. Cross-cultural comparability of quality of life measures. Drug Inf J. 1993;27(2):395-400.

237. Atkinson MJ, Lennox RD. Extending basic principles of measurement models to the design and validation of patient reported outcomes. Health Qual Life Outcomes. 2006;4(1):65.

238. da Mota Falcao D, Ciconelli RM, Ferraz MB. Translation and cultural adaptation of quality of life questionnaires: an evaluation of methodology. J Rheumatol. 2003;30(2):379-85.

239. Herdman M, Fox-Rushby J, Badia X. A model of equivalence in the cultural adaptation of HRQoL instruments: the universalist approach. Qual Life Res. 1998;7(4):323-35.

240. Herdman M, Fox-Rushby J, Badia X. 'Equivalence' and the translation and adaptation of health-related quality of life questionnaires. Qual Life Res. 1997;6(3):237-47.

241. Wild D, Eremenco S, Mear I, Martin M, Houchin C, Gawlicki M, et al. Multinational trials-recommendations on the translations required, approaches to using the same language in different countries, and the approaches to support pooling the data: the ISPOR Patient-Reported Outcomes Translation and Linguistic Validation Good Research Practices Task Force report. Value Health. 2009;12(4):430-40.

242. Wild D, Grove A, Martin M, Eremenco S, Ford S, Verjee-Lorenz A, et al. Principles of good practice for the translation and cultural adaptation process for patient reported outcomes (PRO) measures: report of the ISPOR Task Force for Translation and Cultural Adaptation. Value Health. 2005;8(2):94-104.

243. Acquadro C, Conway K, Hareendran A, Aaronson N. Literature review of methods to translate health-related quality of life questionnaires for use in multinational clinical trials. Value Health. 2008;11(3):509-21.

244. Beaton DE, Bombardier C, Guillemin F, Ferraz MB. Guidelines for the process of cross-cultural adaptation of self-report measures. Spine (Phila Pa 1976). 2000;25(24):3186-91.

245. Dewolf L, Koller M, Velikova G, Johnson C, Scott N, Bottomley A. EORTC Quality of Life Group: translation procedure, 3rd ed.; 2009 [cited 2011 November 26]. Available from: http://groups.eortc.be/qol/sites/default/files/archives/translation_manual_2009.pdf

246. Eremenco SL, Cella D, Arnold BJ. A comprehensive method for the translation and cross-cultural validation of health status questionnaires. Eval Health Prof. 2005;28(2):212-32.

247. Sperber AD. Translation and validation of study instruments for cross-cultural research. Gastroenterology. 2004;126(1 Suppl 1):S124-8.

248. Ware JE, Jr., Keller SD, Gandek B, Brazier JE, Sullivan M. Evaluating translations of health status questionnaires. Methods from the IQOLA project. International Quality of Life Assessment. Int J Technol Assess Health Care. 1995;11(3):525-51.

249. Centers for Disease Control and Prevention. Prevalence and most common causes of disability among adults - United States, 2005. MMWR Morbidity and Mortality Weekly Report. 2009;58(16):421-6.

250. National Council on Disability. The current state of health care for people with disabilities. Washington, DC: National Council on Disability; 2009. Available from: http://purl.fdlp.gov/GPO/gpo3755

251. Agency for Healthcare Research and Quality. Developing quality of care measures for people with disabilities: summary of expert meeting. AHRQ Publication No. 10-0103. Rockville, MD: US Agency for Healthcare Research and Quality; 2010. Available from: http://www.ahrq.gov/populations/devqmdis/.

252. The Center for Universal Design. The principles of universal design, version 2.0. Raleigh, NC: North Carolina State University; 1997. Available from: http://www.ncsu.edu/ncsu/design/cud/about_ud/udprinciples.htm.

253. Story MF. Maximizing usability: the principles of universal design. Assist Technol. 1998;10(1):4-12.

254. Section 508 of the Rehabilitation Act, as amended by the Workforce Investment Act of 1998 (P.L. 105-220) 1998 [cited 2010]. Available from: http://www.section508.gov/.

255. Harniss M, Amtmann D, Cook D, Johnson K. Considerations for developing interfaces for collecting patient-reported outcomes that allow the inclusion of individuals with disabilities. Med Care. 2007;45(5 Suppl 1):S48-S54.

256. Schwartz CE, Sprangers MA. Methodological approaches for assessing response shift in longitudinal health-related quality-of-life research. Soc Sci Med. 1999;48(11):1531-48.

257. Nolte S, Elsworth GR, Sinclair AJ, Osborne RH. Tests of measurement invariance failed to support the application of the "then-test". J Clin Epidemiol. 2009;62(11):1173-80.

258. Cella D, Hahn EA, Dineen K. Meaningful change in cancer-specific quality of life scores: differences between improvement and worsening. Qual Life Res. 2002;11(3):207-21.

259. Brossart DF, Clay DL, Willson VL. Methodological and statistical considerations for threats to internal validity in pediatric outcome data: response shift in self-report outcomes. J Pediatr Psychol. 2002;27(1):97-107.

260. Schwartz CE. Applications of response shift theory and methods to participation measurement: a brief history of a young field. Arch Phys Med Rehabil. 2010;91(9 Suppl):S38-43.

261. Ring L, Hofer S, Heuston F, Harris D, O'Boyle CA. Response shift masks the treatment impact on patient reported outcomes (PROs): the example of individual quality of life in edentulous patients. Health Qual Life Outcomes. 2005;3:55.

262. Ahmed S, Bourbeau J, Maltais F, Mansour A. The Oort structural equation modeling approach detected a response shift after a COPD self-management program not detected by the Schmitt technique. J Clin Epidemiol. 2009;62(11):1165-72.

263. Mayo NE, Scott SC, Ahmed S. Case management poststroke did not induce response shift: the value of residuals. J Clin Epidemiol. 2009;62(11):1148-56.

264. Ramachandran S, Lundy JJ, Coons SJ. Testing the measurement equivalence of paper and touch-screen versions of the EQ-5D visual analog scale (EQ VAS). Qual Life Res. 2008;17(8):1117-20.

265. Dillman DA, Smyth JD, Christian LM. Internet, mail, and mixed-mode surveys: the tailored design method. Hoboken, NJ: Wiley; 2009.

266. Troxel AB, Fairclough DL, Curran D, Hahn EA. Statistical analysis of quality of life with missing data in cancer clinical trials. Stat Med. 1998;17(5-7):653-66.

267. Little RJA, Rubin DB. Statistical Analysis with Missing Data. Hoboken, NJ: Wiley; 2002.

268. Keeter S, Kennedy C, Dimock M, Best J, Craighill P. Gauging the impact of growing nonresponse on estimates from a national RDD telephone survey. Public Opin Q. 2006;70(5):759-79.

269. Johnson TP, Wislar JS. Response rates and nonresponse errors in surveys. JAMA. 2012;307(17):1805-6.

270. Johnson TP, Holbrook AL, Ik Cho Y, Bossarte RM. Nonresponse error in injury-risk surveys. Am J Prev Med. 2006;31(5):427-36.

271. Cull WL, O'Connor KG, Sharp S, Tang S-fS. Response rates and response bias for 50 surveys of pediatricians. Health Serv Res. 2005;40(1):213-26.

272. Purdie DM, Dunne MP, Boyle FM, Cook MD, Najman JM. Health and demographic characteristics of respondents in an Australian national sexuality survey: comparison with population norms. J Epidemiol Community Health. 2002;56(10):748-53.

273. Voigt LF, Koepsell TD, Daling JR. Characteristics of telephone survey respondents according to willingness to participate. Am J Epidemiol. 2003;157(1):66-73.

274. Fairclough DL. Design and analysis of quality of life studies in clinical trials. Boca Raton, FL: Chapman & Hall/CRC Press; 2002.

275. Little RA. Modeling the drop-out mechanism in repeated-measures studies. J Am Statist Assoc. 1995;90(431):1112-21.

276. Littell RC, Milliken GA, Stroup WW, Wolfinger RD. SAS System for MIXED Models. Cary, NC: SAS Institute, Inc.; 1996.

277. Hahn EA, Glendenning GA, Sorensen MV, Hudgens SA, Druker BJ, Guilhot F, et al. Quality of life in patients with newly diagnosed chronic phase chronic myeloid leukemia on imatinib versus interferon alfa plus low-dose cytarabine: results from the IRIS Study. J Clin Oncol. 2003;21(11):2138-46.

278. Fairclough DL, Peterson HF, Cella D, Bonomi P. Comparison of several model-based methods for analysing incomplete quality of life data in cancer clinical trials. Stat Med. 1998;17(5-7):781-96.

279. Basch EM, Reeve BB, Mitchell SA, Clauser SB, Minasian L, Sit L, et al. Electronic toxicity monitoring and patient-reported outcomes. Cancer J. 2011;17(4):231-4.

280. Guyatt G, Schunemann H. How can quality of life researchers make their work more useful to health workers and their patients? Qual Life Res. 2007;16(7):1097-105.

281. Revicki DA, Osoba D, Fairclough D, Barofsky I, Berzon R, Leidy NK, et al. Recommendations on health-related quality of life research to support labeling and promotional claims in the United States. Qual Life Res. 2000;9(8):887-900.

282. Deyo RA, Patrick DL. Barriers to the use of health status measures in clinical investigation, patient care, and policy research. Med Care. 1989;27(3 Suppl):S254-68.

283. Lipscomb J, Donaldson MS, Arora NK, Brown ML, Clauser SB, Potosky AL, et al. Cancer outcomes research. J Natl Cancer Inst Monogr. 2004(33):178-97.

284. Snyder CF, Aaronson NK, Choucair AK, Elliott TE, Greenhalgh J, Halyard MY, et al. Implementing patient-reported outcomes assessment in clinical practice: a review of the options and considerations. Qual Life Res. 2011:S76–S85.

285. Mokkink LB, Terwee CB, Patrick DL, Alonso J, Stratford PW, Knol DL, et al. The COSMIN study reached international consensus on taxonomy, terminology, and definitions of measurement properties for health-related patient-reported outcomes. J Clin Epidemiol. 2010;63(7):737-45.

286. Revicki DA, Gnanasakthy A, Weinfurt K. Documenting the rationale and psychometric characteristics of patient reported outcomes for labeling and promotional claims: the PRO Evidence Dossier. Qual Life Res. 2007;16(4):717-23.

287. Schunemann HJ, Akl EA, Guyatt GH. Interpreting the results of patient reported outcome measures in clinical trials: the clinician's perspective. Health Qual Life Outcomes. 2006;4:62.

288. Butt Z, Reeve B. Enhancing the patient's voice: standards in the design and selection of patient-reported outcomes measures (PROMs) for use in patient-centered outcomes research 2012 [cited 2012 June 15]. Available from: http://www.pcori.org/assets/Enhancing-the-Patients-Voice-Standards-in-the-Design-and-Selection-of-Patient-Reported-Outcomes-Measures-for-Use-in-Patient-Centered-Outcomes-Research.pdf.

289. US Food and Drug Administration (FDA), Center for Drug Evaluation and Research, Center for Biologics Evaluation and Research, Center for Devices and Radiological Health. Guidance for industry patient-reported outcome measures: use in medical product development to support labeling claims. Rockville, MD: FDA; 2009. Available from: http://purl.access.gpo.gov/GPO/LPS113413.

290. US Food and Drug Administration. Draft guidance for industry. Qualification process for drug development tools 2010 [cited 2014 June 30]. Available from: http://www.fda.gov/downloads/Drugs/GuidanceComplianceRegulatoryInformation/Guidances/UCM230597.pdf.

291. Erickson P, Willke R, Burke L. A concept taxonomy and an instrument hierarchy: tools for establishing and evaluating the conceptual framework of a patient-reported outcome (PRO) instrument as applied to product labeling claims. Value Health. 2009;12(8):1158-67.

292. Patrick DL, Burke LB, Powers JH, Scott JA, Rock EP, Dawisha S, et al. Patient-reported outcomes to support medical product labeling claims: FDA perspective. Value Health. 2007;10 Suppl 2:S125-37.

293. Scientific Advisory Committee of the Medical Outcomes Trust. Assessing health status and quality of life instruments: attributes and review criteria. Qual Life Res. 2002(11):193-205.

294. Mokkink LB, Terwee CB, Gibbons E, Stratford PW, Alonso J, Patrick DL, et al. Inter-rater agreement and reliability of the COSMIN (COnsensus-based Standards for the selection of health status Measurement INstruments) checklist. BMC Med Res Methodol. 2010;10:82.

295. Angst F. The new COSMIN guidelines confront traditional concepts of responsiveness. BMC Med Res Methodol. 2011;11(1):152.

296. Mokkink LB, Terwee CB, Knol DL, Stratford PW, Alonso J, Patrick DL, et al. The COSMIN checklist for evaluating the methodological quality of studies on measurement properties: a clarification of its content. BMC Med Res Methodol. 2010;10:22.

297. Mokkink LB, Terwee CB, Patrick DL, Alonso J, Stratford PW, Knol DL, et al. The COSMIN checklist for assessing the methodological quality of studies on measurement properties of health status measurement instruments: an international Delphi study. Qual Life Res. 2010;19(4):539-49.

298. Terwee CB, Mokkink LB, Knol DL, Ostelo RW, Bouter LM, de Vet HC. Rating the methodological quality in systematic reviews of studies on measurement properties: a scoring system for the COSMIN checklist. Qual Life Res. 2011;21(4):651-7.

299. Johnson C, Aaronson N, Blazeby JM, Bottomley A, Fayers P, Koller M, et al. EORTC Quality of Life Group: guidelines for developing questionnaire modules 2011, 4th ed. [cited 2011 November 26]. Available from: http://groups.eortc.be/qol/Pdf%20presentations/Guidelines%20for%20 Developing%20questionnaire-%20FINAL.pdf.

300. Rothman M, Burke L, Erickson P, Leidy NK, Patrick DL, Petrie CD. Use of existing patient-reported outcome (PRO) instruments and their modification: the ISPOR Good Research Practices for Evaluating and Documenting Content Validity for the Use of Existing Instruments and Their Modification PRO task force report. Value Health. 2009;12(8):1075-83.

301. Wild D, Grove A, Martin M, Eremenco S, McElroy S, Verjee-Lorenz A, et al. Principles of good practice for the translation and cultural adaptation process for patient-reported outcomes (PRO) measures: report of the ISPOR Task Force for Translation and Cultural Adaptation. Value Health. 2005;8(2):94-104.

302. Magasi S, Ryan G, Revicki D, Lenderking W, Hays RD, Brod M, et al. Content validity of patient-reported outcome measures: perspectives from a PROMIS meeting. Qual Life Res. 2012 Jun;21(5):739-46.

303. Valderas JM, Ferrer M, Mendivil J, Garin O, Rajmil L, Herdman M, et al. Development of EMPRO: a tool for the standardized assessment of patient-reported outcome measures. Value Health. 2008;11(4):700-8.

304. Revicki D, Hays RD, Cella D, Sloan J. Recommended methods for determining responsiveness and minimally important differences for patient-reported outcomes. J Clin Epidemiol. 2008;61(2):102-9.

305. Ahmed S, Berzon RA, Revicki DA, Lenderking WR, Moinpour CM, Basch E, et al. The use of patient-reported outcomes (PRO) within comparative effectiveness research: implications for clinical practice and health care policy. Med Care. 2012;50(12):1060-70.

306. PROMIS Validity Standards Committee on behalf of the PROMIS Network of investigators. The PROMIS instrument development and psychometric evaluation scientific standards. 2012.

307. Bellamy N. WOMAC Osteoarthritis Index: user guide IX. Brisbane: Nicholas Bellamy; 2008.

308. Bellamy N, Buchanan WW. A preliminary evaluation of the dimensionality and clinical importance of pain and disability in osteoarthritis of the hip and knee. Clin Rheumatol. 1986;5(2):231-41.

309. Pua YH, Cowan SM, Wrigley TV, Bennell KL. Discriminant validity of the Western Ontario and McMaster Universities Osteoarthritis Index Physical Functioning Subscale in community samples with hip osteoarthritis. Arch Phys Med Rehabil. 2009;90(10):1772-7.

310. Bellamy N, Buchanan WW, Goldsmith CH, Campbell J, Stitt LW. Validation study of WOMAC: a health status instrument for measuring clinically important patient relevant outcomes to antirheumatic drug therapy in patients with osteoarthritis of the hip or knee. J Rheumatol. 1988;15(12):1833-40.

311. Dunbar MJ, Robertsson O, Ryd L, Lidgren L. Appropriate questionnaires for knee arthroplasty. Results of a survey of 3600 patients from the Swedish Knee Arthroplasty Registry. J Bone Joint Surg Br. 2001;83(3):339-44.

312. McConnell S, Kolopack P, Davis AM. The Western Ontario and McMaster Universities Osteoarthritis Index (WOMAC): a review of its utility and measurement properties. Arthritis Rheum. 2001;45(5):453-61.

313. Bullens P, van Loon C, de Waal Malefijt M, Laan R, Veth R. Patient satisfaction after total knee arthroplasty. J Arthroplasty. 2001;16(6):740-7.

314. Robertsson O, Dunbar MJ. Patient satisfaction compared with general health and disease-specific questionnaires in knee arthroplasty patients. J Arthroplasty. 2001;16(4):476-82.

315. Brazier JE, Harper R, Munro J, Walters SJ, Snaith ML. Generic and condition-specific outcome measures for people with osteoarthritis of the knee. Rheumatology. 1999;38(9):870-7.

316. Davies GM, Watson DJ, Bellamy N. Comparison of the responsiveness and relative effect size of the Western Ontario and McMaster Universities Osteoarthritis Index and the short-form Medical Outcomes Study Survey in a randomized, clinical trial of osteoarthritis patients. Arthritis Care Res. 1999;12(3):172-9.

317. Dworkin RH, Turk DC, Wyrwich KW, Beaton D, Cleeland CS, Farrar JT, et al. Interpreting the clinical importance of treatment outcomes in chronic pain clinical trials: IMMPACT recommendations. J Pain. 2008;9(2):105-21.

318. Bellamy N, Wilson C, Hendrikz J. Population-based normative values for the Western Ontario and McMaster (WOMAC) Osteoarthritis Index: part I. Semin Arthritis Rheum. 2011;41(2):139-48.

319. Tubach F, Ravaud P, Baron G, Falissard B, Logeart I, Bellamy N, et al. Evaluation of clinically relevant changes in patient reported outcomes in knee and hip osteoarthritis: the minimal clinically important improvement. Ann Rheum Dis. 2005;64(1):29-33.

320. Marshall D, Pericak D, Grootendorst P, Gooch K, Faris P, Frank C, et al. Validation of a prediction model to estimate health utilities index Mark 3 utility scores from WOMAC index scores in patients with osteoarthritis of the hip. Value Health. 2008;11(3):470-7.

321. Tubach F, Baron G, Falissard B, Logeart I, Dougados M, Bellamy N, et al. Using patients' and rheumatologists' opinions to specify a short form of the WOMAC function subscale. Ann Rheum Dis. 2005;64(1):75-9.

322. Bellamy N, Patel B, Davis T, Dennison S. Electronic data capture using the Womac NRS 3.1 Index (m-Womac): a pilot study of repeated independent remote data capture in OA. Inflammopharmacology. 2010;18(3):107-11.

323. Bellamy N, Wilson C, Hendrikz J, Whitehouse SL, Patel B, Dennison S, et al. Osteoarthritis Index delivered by mobile phone (m-WOMAC) is valid, reliable, and responsive. J Clin Epidemiol. 2011;64(2):182-90.

324. Theiler R, Bischoff-Ferrari HA, Good M, Bellamy N. Responsiveness of the electronic touch screen WOMAC 3.1 OA Index in a short term clinical trial with rofecoxib. Osteoarthritis Cartilage. 2004;12(11):912-6.

325. American College of Rheumatology. Western Ontario and McMaster Universities Osteoarthritis Index (WOMAC) 2011 [updated 2012; cited 2012 July 6]. Available from: http://www.rheumatology.org/practice/clinical/clinicianresearchers/outcomes-instrumentation/WOMAC.asp.

326. Kazis LE, Miller DR, Skinner KM, Lee A, Ren XS, Clark JA, et al. Applications of methodologies of the Veterans Health Study in the VA healthcare system: conclusions and summary. J Ambul Care Manage. 2006;29(2):182-8.

327. Kazis LE, Selim A, Rogers W, Ren XS, Lee A, Miller DR. Dissemination of methods and results from the Veterans Health Study: final comments and implications for future monitoring strategies within and outside the veterans healthcare system. J Ambul Care Manage. 2006;29(4):310-9.

328. Haffer SC, Bowen SE. Measuring and improving health outcomes in Medicare: the Medicare HOS program. Health Care Financ Rev. 2004;25(4):1-3.

329. National Committee for Quality Assurance, Committee on Performance Measurement. HEDIS 2006: health plan employer data & information set. Washington, DC: National Committee for Quality Assurance; 2006.

330. Jordan JE, Osborne RH, Buchbinder R. Critical appraisal of health literacy indices revealed variable underlying constructs, narrow content and psychometric weaknesses. J Clin Epidemiol. 2011;64(4):366-79.

331. Cella D, Nowinski C. Measuring quality of life in chronic illness: the functional assessment of chronic illness therapy measurement system. Arch Phys Med Rehabil. 2002;83(Suppl. 2):S10-S7.

332. FDA Center for Drug Evaluation and Research Quality of Life Subcommittee, Oncologic Drugs Advisory Committee. Background letter. Bethesda, MD: US Food and Drug Administration; 2000 Feb 10. Available from: http://www.fda.gov/ohrms/dockets/ac/00/backgrd/3591b1a.pdf.

333. Shearer D, Morshed S. Common generic measures of health related quality of life in injured patients. Injury. 2011;42(3):241-7.

334. Owolabi MO. Which is more valid for stroke patients: generic or stroke-specific quality of life measures? Neuroepidemiology. 2010;34(1):8-12.

335. Bergland A, Thorsen H, Kåresen R. Association between generic and disease-specific quality of life questionnaires and mobility and balance among women with osteoporosis and vertebral fractures. Aging Clin Exp Res. 2011;23(4):296-303.

336. Rothrock N, Hays R, Spritzer K, Yount SE, Riley W, Cella D. Relative to the general US population, chronic diseases are associated with poorer health-related quality of life as measured by the Patient-Reported Outcomes Measurement Information System (PROMIS). J Clin Epidemiol. 2010;63(11):1195-204.

337. Chakravarty EF, Bjorner JB, Fries JF. Improving patient reported outcomes using item response theory and computerized adaptive testing. J Rheumatol. 2007;34(6):1426-31.

338. Donaldson G. Patient-reported outcomes and the mandate of measurement. Qual Life Res. 2008;17(10):1303-13.

339. Lai JS, Cella D, Choi SW, Junghaenel DU, Christodolou C, Gershon R, et al. How item banks and their application can influence measurement practice in rehabilitation medicine: a PROMIS Fatigue Item Bank example. Arch Phys Med Rehabil. 2011;92(10 Suppl):S20-S7.

340. Rose M, Bjorner JB, Becker J, Fries JF, Ware JE. Evaluation of a preliminary physical function item bank supported the expected advantages of the Patient-Reported Outcomes Measurement Information System (PROMIS). J Clin Epidemiol. 2008;61(1):17-33.

341. Kirshner B, Guyatt G. A methodological framework for assessing health indices. J Chronic Dis. 1985;38(1):27-36.

342. McClendon DT, Warren JS, Green KM, Burlingame GM, Eggett DL, McClendon RJ. Sensitivity to change of youth treatment outcome measures: a comparison of the CBCL, BASC-2, and Y-OQ. J Clin Psychol. 2011;67(1):111-25.

343. Terwee CB, Dekker FW, Wiersinga WM, Prummel MF, Bossuyt PM. On assessing responsiveness of health-related quality of life instruments: guidelines for instrument evaluation. Qual Life Res. 2003;12(4):349-62.

344. Beaton DE, van Eerd D, Smith P, van der Velde G, Cullen K, Kennedy CA, et al. Minimal change is sensitive, less specific to recovery: a diagnostic testing approach to interpretability. J Clin Epidemiol. 2011;64(5):487-96.

345. Andresen EM, Meyers AR. Health-related quality of life outcomes measures. Arch Phys Med Rehabil. 2000;81(12 Suppl 2):S30-45.

346. Vermeersch DA, Lambert MJ, Burlingame GM. Outcome questionnaire: item sensitivity to change. J Pers Assess. 2000;74(2):242-61.

347. Shikiar R, Willian MK, Okun MM, Thompson CS, Revicki DA. The validity and responsiveness of three quality of life measures in the assessment of psoriasis patients: results of a phase II study. Health Qual Life Outcomes. 2006;4:71.

348. Schroter S, Lamping DL. Responsiveness of the coronary revascularisation outcome questionnaire compared with the SF-36 and Seattle Angina Questionnaire. Qual Life Res. 2006;15(6):1069-78.

349. Kaplan RM, Tally S, Hays RD, Feeny D, Ganiats TG, Palta M, et al. Five preference-based indexes in cataract and heart failure patients were not equally responsive to change. J Clin Epidemiol. 2011;64(5):497-506.

350. Bauer S, Lambert MJ, Nielsen SL. Clinical significance methods: a comparison of statistical techniques. J Pers Assess. 2004;82(1):60-70.

351. Crosby RD, Kolotkin RL, Williams GR. Defining clinically meaningful change in health-related quality of life. Jouornal of Clinical Epidemiology. 2003;56(5):395-407.

352. Brozek JL, Guyatt GH, Schunemann HJ. How a well-grounded minimal important difference can enhance transparency of labelling claims and improve interpretation of a patient reported outcome measure. Health Qual Life Outcomes. 2006;4(69):1-7

353. Jaeschke R, Singer J, Guyatt GH. Measurement of health status. Ascertaining the minimal clinically important difference. Control Clin Trials. 1989;10(4):407-15.

354. Lydick E, Epstein RS. Interpretation of quality of life changes. Qual Life Res. 1993;2(3):221-6.

355. Revicki D, Hays R, Cella D, Sloan J. Recommended methods for determining responsiveness and minimally important differences for patient-reported outcomes. J Clin Epidemiol. 2008;61(2):102-9.

356. Farivar SS, Liu H, Hays RD. Half standard deviation estimate of the minimally important difference in HRQOL scores? Expert Rev Pharmacoecon Outcomes Res. 2004;4(5):515-23.

357. Guyatt GH. Making sense of quality-of-life data. Med Care. 2000;38(9 Suppl):II175-9.

358. Guyatt GH, Norman GR, Juniper EF, Griffith LE. A critical look at transition ratings. J Clin Epidemiol. 2002;55(9):900-8.

359. Rejas J, Pardo A, Ruiz MA. Standard error of measurement as a valid alternative to minimally important difference for evaluating the magnitude of changes in patient-reported outcomes measures. J Clin Epidemiol. 2008;61(4):350-6.

360. Norman G, Sloan J, Wyrwich K. Interpretation of changes in health-related quality of life: the remarkable universality of half a standard deviation. Med Care. 2003;41(5):582-92.

361. Chaudhry B, Wang J, Wu S, Maglione M, Mojica W, Roth E, et al. Systematic review: impact of health information technology on quality, efficiency, and costs of medical care. Ann Intern Med. 2006;144(10):742-52.

362. Goldzweig CL, Maglione M, Shekelle PG, Towfigh A. Costs and benefits of health information technology: New trends from the literature. Health Aff (Millwood). 2009;28(2):w282-w93.

363. Wilson EV. Patient-centered e-health. Hershey, PA: Medical Information Science Reference; 2009.

364. Harris Interactive, ARiA Marketing. Healthcare satisfaction study. Rochester, NY: Harris Interactive; 2000.

365. Davis F. User acceptance of information technology: system characteristics, user perceptions and behavioral impacts. Int J Man Mach Stud. 1993;38(3):475-87.

366. US Department of Health and Human Services, Office of the National Coordinator for Health Information Technology. Meaningful use 2011 [cited 2011 July]. Available from: http://healthit.hhs.gov/portal/server.pt?open=512&objID=2996&mode=2.

367. Estabrooks PA, Boyle M, Emmons KM, Glasgow RE, Hesse BW, Kaplan RM, et al. Harmonized patient-reported data elements in the electronic health record: supporting meaningful use by primary care action on health behaviors and key psychosocial factors. J Am Med Inform Assoc. 2012;19(4):575-82.

368. Bitton A, Flier LA, Jha AK. Health information technology in the era of care delivery reform: to what end? JAMA. 2012;307(24):2593-4.

369. Adler-Milstein J, Jha AK. Sharing clinical data electronically: a critical challenge for fixing the health care system. JAMA. 2012;307(16):1695-6.

370. Masys D, Baker D, Butros A, Cowles KE. Giving patients access to their medical records via the internet: the PCASSO experience. J Am Med Inform Assoc. 2002;9(2):181-91.

371. Nelson EC, Hvitfeldt H, Reid RM, Grossman D, Lindblad S, Mastanduno MP, et al. Using patient-reported information to improve health outcomes and health care value: case studies from Dartmouth, Karolinska and Group Health. Technical report. Lebanon, NH: Dartmouth Institute for Health Policy and Clinical Practice, 2012.

372. Davis K, Yount S, Del Ciello K, Whalen M, Khan S, Bass M, et al. An innovative symptom monitoring tool for people with advanced lung cancer: a pilot demonstration. J Support Oncol. 2007;5(8):381-7.

373. Harris WH, Sledge CB. Total hip and total knee replacement (1). N Engl J Med. 1990;323(11):725-31.

374. Harris WH, Sledge CB. Total hip and total knee replacement (2). N Engl J Med. 1990;323(12):801-7.

375. Liang MH, Cullen KE, Poss R. Primary total hip or knee replacement: evaluation of patients. Ann Intern Med. 1982;97(5):735-9.

376. Kroll MA, Otis JC, Sculco TP, Lee AC, Paget SA, Bruckenstein R, et al. The relationship of stride characteristics to pain before and after total knee arthroplasty. Clin Orthop Relat Res. 1989(239):191-5.

377. Ethgen O, Bruyère O, Richy F, Dardennes C, Reginster JY. Health-related quality of life in total hip and total knee arthroplasty. A qualitative and systematic review of the literature. J Bone Joint Join Surg Am. 2004; 86-A(5):86.

378. Birrell F, Johnell O, Silman A. Projecting the need for hip replacement over the next three decades: influence of changing demography and threshold for surgery. Ann Rheum Dis. 1999;58(9):569-72.

379. Rissanen P, Aro S, Sintonen H, Asikainen K, Slätis P, Paavolainen P. Costs and cost-effectiveness in hip and knee replacements. A prospective study. Int J Technol Assess Health Care. 1997;13(4):575-88.

380. Williams MH, Newton JN, Frankel SJ, Braddon F, Barclay E, Gray JAM. Prevalence of total hip replacement: how much demand has been met? J Epidemiol Community Health. 1994;48(2):188-91.

Acknowledgments

The authors thank Kathleen Swantek, MLIS, for assistance with reference management. We also acknowledge our appreciation for helpful comments on the content of an earlier draft of this work from Karen Adams, PhD, MT; Ethan Basch, MD, MSc; Victor Chang, MD; Stephan Fihn, MD, MPH; Floyd Jackson Fowler, PhD; Lewis Kazis, ScD; Jennifer Moore; Eugene Nelson, DSc, MPH; Kenneth Ottenbacher, PhD, OTR; Karen Pace, PhD, MSN; and Mary Tinetti, MD. We also acknowledge the expert assistance of Joanne Studders, BA, and Loraine Monroe for diligent editing and document preparation, respectively.

About the Authors

Zeeshan Butt, PhD, is an Associate Professor of Medical Social Sciences, Surgery, and Psychiatry and Behavioral Sciences at Northwestern University Feinberg School of Medicine. He also serves as the Associate Director of the Center for Patient-Centered Outcomes there.

David Cella, PhD, is a Professor and Chair of the Department of Medical Social Sciences at Northwestern University Feinberg School of Medicine. He is the principal investigator of the National Institutes of Health (NIH) Initiative "HealthMeasures: A Person-Centered Assessment System," which curates and distributes PROMIS (the Patient Reported Outcomes Measurement Information System) and three other health measurement systems. Dr. Cella is also a founding member and officer of the PROMIS Health Organization, a charitable organization that licenses and promotes the use of PROMIS worldwide.

Elizabeth A. Hahn, MA, is an Associate Professor in the Departments of Medical Social Sciences and Preventive Medicine, and the Institute for Public Health and Medicine, at Northwestern University Feinberg School of Medicine. Her research primarily involves patient-reported outcomes in chronic illnesses, with a focus on underserved populations and health disparities.

Sally E. Jensen, PhD, is a Research Assistant Professor in the Departments of Medical Social Sciences and Surgery at Northwestern University Feinberg School of Medicine. Her research focuses on patient-reported outcomes across various medical and surgical patient populations.

Kathleen N. Lohr, PhD, is a Distinguished Fellow at RTI International. Her research has involved comparative effectiveness and evidence-based practice, measurement of health status and quality of life, quality of care assessment, clinical practice guidelines, and related health policy issues.

Cindy J. Nowinski, MD, PhD, is a Research Associate Professor in the Departments of Medical Social Sciences and Neurology at Northwestern University Feinberg School of Medicine. Her research focuses on the development of patient-reported and objective health outcome measures for use in clinical and epidemiological research and clinical care.

Nan Rothrock, PhD, is a Research Associate Professor in the Department of Medical Social Sciences at Northwestern University Feinberg School of Medicine. Her research focuses on development and application of patient-reported outcome measures in research and practice.

Made in the USA
Lexington, KY
16 January 2016